WHY YOUR DOCTOR OFFERS NUTRITIONAL SUPPLEMENTS

REVISED THIRD EDITION

Stephanie Selene Anderson
with Mark R. Anderson

Edits and Revision, Third Edition
Patrick Earvolino

Published by

Selene River Press

Publisher and Distributor of Select Books on Health

P.O. Box 270091
Fort Collins, Colorado 80527
866-407-9323
www.seleneriverpress.com
info@seleneriverpress.com

First edition published 1988. Second edition 2004. Third edition 2010.

Book Design by Brian Gabel
Additional Design for Third Edition by Norm Kitten
Cover Art (front and back) by Ginny Hogan. Copyright © Ginny Hogan
Photographs by Stephanie Selene Anderson
Editorial by Susan Bouse, Bouse Editorial

Note to the Reader*: The ideas and suggestions contained in this book are not intended as a substitute for the appropriate care by a licensed healthcare practitioner.*

ISBN 978-0-9645709-9-3

Printed in the United States of America
10 9 8 7 6 5 4 3 2 1

Acknowledgments

With thanks to the sharp editorial services of Karen Grasso and Jane D. Albritton; the generous consulting services of the perspicacious Judith DeCava; and the hearty support of Kim Knight, Dean Turner, and Jane C. Mirandette. And to Patrick Earvolino for refreshing this third edition with critical updates and revisions.

We are grateful to the gracious Bonnie Antich and Scott LeCocq of Colorado for use of their Canyon Spirit Gallery and Bonnie's beautiful pottery.

Instinct is extinct; but there are those who have kept knowledge extant.

—Mark R. Anderson

With everlasting thanks to Dr. Royal Lee

Table of Contents

Introduction Why We Need Nutritional Supplements

"Can't I get all the nutrients I need from my diet?" It's a question health practitioners hear all the time. Sadly, in today's nutritionally challenged world, the answer to this question is almost certainly "No."

For reasons you will learn in this little book, much of the food we eat today is tragically deficient in the vitamins, minerals, and other nutrients required by the human body. Much of it also contains synthetic chemicals that are toxic to the body. Years of consuming these "counterfeit" foods have put our health behind the eight ball. As a result, we must not only learn to make better food choices, we must also feed our body concentrated, whole-food supplements to get it back on track.

Understanding what makes a food or a supplement good can be a daunting task. Fortunately, you hold in your hands the key to accomplishing that task. *Why Your Doctor Offers Nutritional Supplements* is the first installment in Selene River Press' Quest for Superior Nutrition series, created to provide a reliable overview of human nutrition and practical ways to secure the very best nourishment for you and your family.

In Sections I through IV of the book, we look at the human food supply, both past and present. As you'll see, people could at one time get adequate nourishment from the food they ate. Some Native Americans, for instance, obtained virtually everything their body required from the buffalo they hunted. While we don't have to kill wild beasts to thrive today, in order to optimize our nutrition we do need to show the same intelligence and understanding of food that allowed American Indians to survive with practically no degenerative diseases.

Such an understanding of food begins with a look at the ultimate sources of human nourishment—the sun and the soil. In examining the importance of these two vital factors as well as the effects of modern food processing, you'll see why conventionally grown foods have come to be so nutrient deficient. We'll then examine the Seven Deadly Fallacies of the Western Diet, including the truth about fat, grains, meat, milk, salt, vegetable oils, and sugar, and the role that each of these plays—or doesn't—in the quest for superior nutrition.

In Sections V and VI, we turn our attention to nutritional supplements. You may think that all supplements are the same, yet nothing could be further from the truth. While the vast majority of supplements *are* similar, in that the raw materials of almost all of them are produced by a handful of pharmaceutical companies, the difference between these mass-produced synthetic chemicals and whole-food concentrates is truly a matter of illness or health as far as your body is concerned. You'll discover just why this is so and find answers to some common questions patients have when starting a nutritional supplement program.

All the knowledge in the world about nutrition won't help you if you don't have a healthy digestive system to assimilate the foods and supplements you've wisely selected. That's why in Section VII, you'll learn the basics of the digestive system and what you and your health practitioner can do to get yours into tip-top shape. And, to ensure that you remain in balance once you get there, you'll find in Section VIII a brief overview of the immune system and the nutrients required by each member of this amazing "health alliance" of the body, including the liver, spleen, skin, thymus, and gastrointestinal (GI) tract.

Finally, in Section IX, you'll discover some all-important tips on how to navigate a health food store. Believe it or not, much of the food sold in stores that claim to be dedicated to your health is anything but good for you, and with the information in this final chapter, you'll know just which foods are truly nutritious and which to avoid at all costs.

The health practitioner who recommended *Why Your Doctor Offers Nutritional Supplements* is trained and committed to helping you transform your lifestyle into one that is healthy and productive, no matter what challenges you face. Of course, ultimately the responsibility for taking control of your health lies with you, but with your health practitioner's help and what you learn in these pages, you can create a diet and supplement program that *will* return you to health.

Your quest for superior nutrition begins here.

—Patrick Earvolino
June 2010

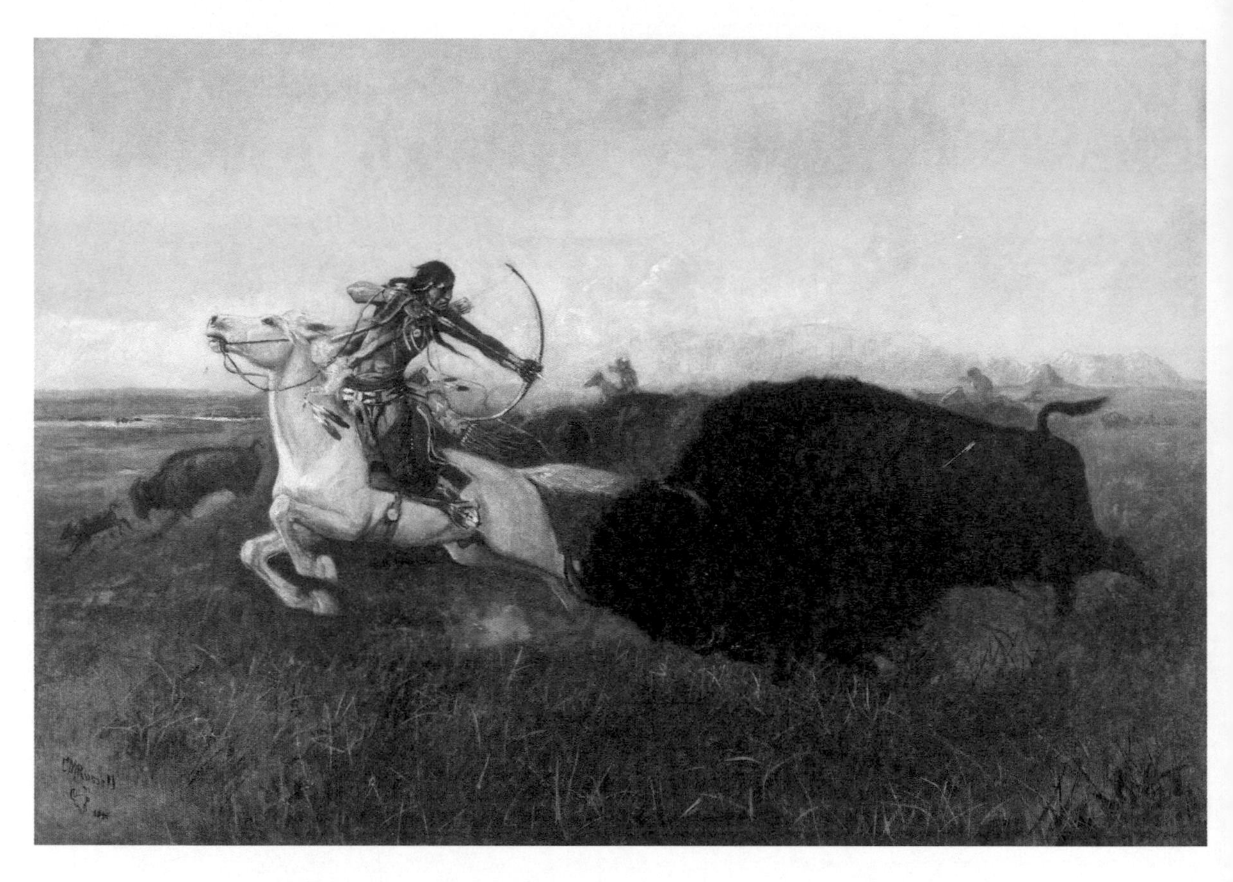

The quest for superior nutrition has never been easy.
(*Indians Hunting Buffalo,* by Charles M. Russell.
Courtesy Sid Richardson Collection of Western Art, Fort Worth, Texas.)

Charles Russell's painting *Indians Hunting Buffalo* powerfully captures the sense of an uncertain outcome: Will this man and his family survive in health and strength, or will he and his horse lose their lives in the quest for superior nutrition? Such grave risk was commensurate with the reward of securing the best food possible for his family, for the buffalo provided every nutrient required by the human body, as you can see.

Human Nutrition Derived from the Entire Buffalo

- Vitamin A from the kidney, liver, and fatty tissue to nourish our eyes, skin, lungs, kidneys, digestive tract, and immune system.
- Vitamin B complex from the liver and muscle meats (including thiamin, riboflavin, niacinamide, folic acid, pyridoxine, pantothenic acid, and vitamin B12) for the health of our heart, nerves, brain, blood cells, fetal development, and energy production.
- Vitamin C complex from the adrenal glands for strong bones, teeth, ligaments, tendons, cartilage, and immune function.
- Vitamin D from exposure of cholesterol in the buffalo's skin to sunlight.
- Vitamin E from the organ meats to support our heart, immune system, tissue repair, and endocrine system.
- Vitamin F from organ fats (including essential omega 3 and 6 fatty acids, healthful saturated fats, and cholesterol) to protect cell membranes and thus support a strong heart and healthy skin, hair, liver, gallbladder, endocrine glands, lymphatic circulation, respiratory tract, and brain.
- Vitamin K from liver for the health of our blood and bones.
- Protein from muscle and organ meats to provide all eight essential amino acids as well as a full spectrum of nonessential aminos, and to act as a source of glucose for energy.
- Iron from organ meats, especially liver, for healthy hemoglobin in our red blood cells—essential for oxygen-rich blood.
- Nucleic acids (RNA and DNA), protomorphogens, and cell determinants from organ meats and marrow for the health of our brain and for organ and tissue repair.
- Enzymes for digestion and immune function and endocrine support from organs.
- Amino acids, collagen, calcium, and other minerals obtained by simmering the buffalo's bones in a soup stock to yield nutrient-rich gelatin, which helps create strong connective tissues such as cartilage and ligaments to ensure stable joints. Soups made from bones also help heal the GI tract by supplying hydrophilic colloids—gelatinous substances that manage water content in the tract.
- In addition, minerals from organ meats and bone soups, including highly absorbable forms of calcium, phosphorus, magnesium, manganese, zinc, iron, copper, selenium, sodium, potassium, and others, also provide essential support to every system and tissue in the human body, including the nervous, skeletal, circulatory, endocrine, respiratory, skin, and immune systems, and form the basis, in conjunction with amino acids, for hundreds of essential enzymes.

...And the buffalo made all this out of grass and water.

To hunt buffalo successfully—to obtain superior nutrition—the American Indian had to summon courage, skill, instinct, intelligence, and knowledge of the characteristics and properties of his food supply. He had to risk life and limb, traveling days or even months from his family and community in order to obtain the very best nutrition.

Today, we've ingeniously developed means to free ourselves from such risks and labors in obtaining food. But in the process, we've lost sight of the goal of the hunt: superior nutrition. We've allowed ourselves to settle for far less than what the American Indian enjoyed, and we are paying dearly for it with our health. We must now exercise the mental equivalent of the American Indian's labor and show the same strength of will, knowledge, and concern in order to achieve our own quest for superior nutrition.

That quest begins with an understanding of our food. Unfortunately, the modern food supply falls far short of providing all that is necessary to produce robust, healthy people. We no longer live in a society that teaches children which foods and methods of preparation will provide superior nutrition. Consequently, many of us are trying to find a new way to educate ourselves and our families about nutrition.

We've all tried turning to doctors for help, but often the doctor or health professional does not have sufficient time or knowledge. And though there is no lack of written information on health and nutrition to turn to in lieu of professional help, without an awareness of the difference between counterfeit and authentic food, or a basic understanding of why the body does not thrive on counterfeit food, it is difficult to discern which information is accurate.

Why Your Doctor Offers Nutritional Supplements was created to assist you in this task. The information in the following pages represents not some new fad diet, but rather a fundamental understanding of the link between human health and nutrition. As you'll see, this connection rests on the health of the soil, plants, and animals of our planet, yet it begins with the source that makes all life possible—the sun.

Section II The Sun: Source of All Energy

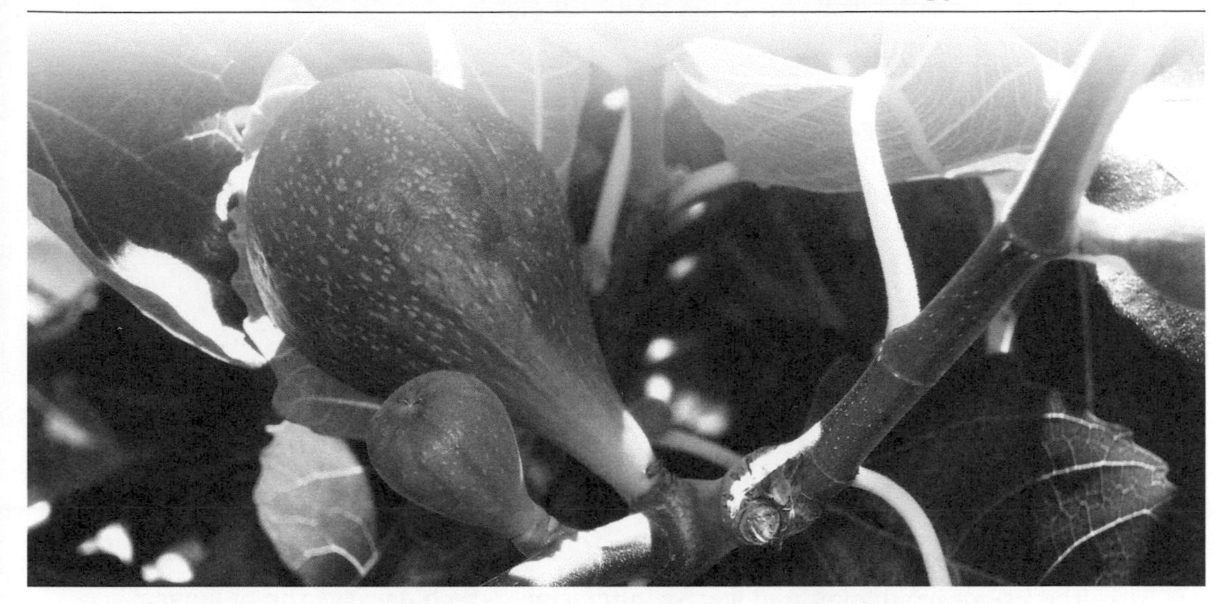

Health results from a balanced flow of life energy, and nutrition plays *the* key role in the production and management of that energy. Why? Because all energy on Earth originates from the sun, and nutrition is how we make that energy available to us.

Humans and animals can't utilize the sun's energy directly, but plants can. Plants convert the sun's energy into nutrients, which we in turn use to feed the powerhouses of our cells—the mitochondria—to produce energy for our body. In the words of the great Dr. Royal Lee:

> The plant lives by absorbing energy from the sun, then using that energy to covert inorganic substances from the soil into organic substances. It converts minerals [and] gases of the air (carbon dioxide and oxygen) into food. The energy is the sun's heat. Your temperature of 98 degrees is the sun's heat stored up by a plant for you to release when you eat that plant.[1]

The sun's energy is stored in the plant along with phytochemicals—complex chemicals made by the plant. Sometimes we liberate the energy and phytochemicals directly by eating and digesting the plant. Other times, we do so indirectly, by eating animals that eat the plants. That's why Dr. Lee liked to say, "When you order a steak, you're eating grass."[2]

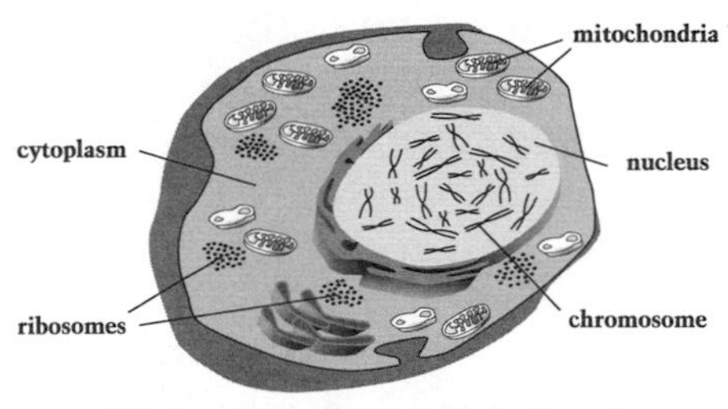

Mitochondria produce energy for the cell through cellular respiration.

The powerful transformation of solar energy to Earth energy is rarely appreciated as the foundation for health. We often hear, "To improve your health, eat a good diet," but this is not much help without an understanding of how the sun's energy is converted into the foods of a superior diet. Instead, the very word "diet" has come to mean whatever is being promoted

---

[1] *Lectures of Dr. Royal Lee, Vol. II.* See Appendix, Audio CDs section.

[2] For a brief biography of Dr. Lee, see About Dr. Royal Lee on p. 55.

as the latest fad for weight loss. We have lost our instinct and knowledge of the best way to access the power of the sun through a healthful diet.

What Is a Good Diet?

According to the U.S. Department of Agriculture, the typical American will consume calories generated from about 50 tons of food in a lifetime. Over 50 percent of those calories will come from refined sugars and altered, synthetic fats—substances a far cry from the plants they were derived from. In fact, most of the foods in today's market are devitalized, demineralized versions of natural plant foods and their precious phytochemicals.

The reasons for this devitalization are many, including:

- farming methods that do not rejuvenate the soil
- chemical farming techniques that contaminate and sterilize the soil
- refining methods that remove or destroy nutrients from food
- the use of chemical preservatives, artificial colors, and flavors that pollute food
- the use of irradiation and genetic alteration, which damage the biological structure of food
- the creation of manmade, junk nonfoods that substitute for healthy food
- the use of agricultural and industrial toxins that contaminate food through pollution of water, air, and land

After eating the "counterfeit" foods resulting from such processes for so many years, it is no surprise that many of us are in ill health. To turn things around, we need to (1) replace counterfeit refined foods with real, nutrient-rich foods, (2) get therapeutic nutritional support to restore proper function to all the body's systems, and (3) develop the ability to recognize truly healthful food.

Why Can't I Live in Wellness?

We know that machine parts wear out or break down from use, neglect, or abuse. But unlike a machine, the human body can renew and regenerate itself—if it has what it needs. The body produces new cells every day for every organ and gland. Healing of injuries, both minor and severe, is routine. Why, then, is health so elusive?

The answer to this question lies beneath our feet. *It is from the soil that plants take up and transform elements into the nutrients we require.* If this foundation of the body's building material and energy is not balanced and consistent, our bodies wear out and break down prematurely. Unfortunately, our modern mechanized world emphasizes quantity rather than quality of foodstuffs. Although we in America pride ourselves on caloric abundance, it's been demonstrated that empty calories and demineralized foods lead to malnutrition just as surely as no food at all.

Sir Robert McCarrison and the Plant-Soil Connection

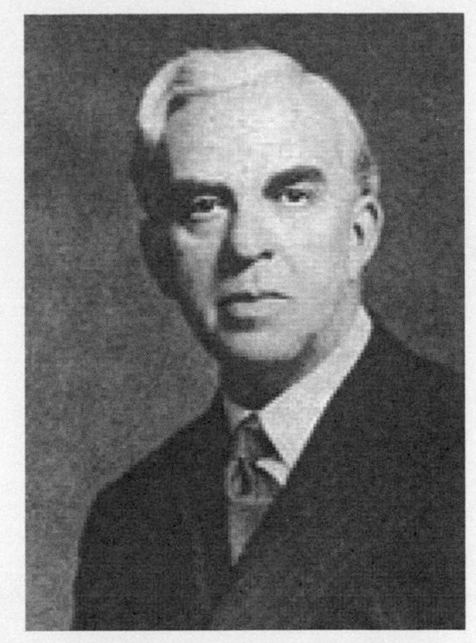

In 1913, when Major General Sir Robert McCarrison, MD, became chief medical officer to the British troops in India, he was already a celebrated endocrine researcher, noted for his discoveries of the cause of goiter. In India, McCarrison would conduct large-scale food experiments on animals and present the first scientific evidence that the endocrine system suffers the first lesions of malnutrition (beginning with the adrenals, then the thymus, then the thyroid), leading to degeneration throughout the body. For his work, McCarrison would be knighted, and in 1928, he became Director of Nutritional Research in India.

McCarrison came to many of his conclusions by studying the Hunzas, a famously healthy people living in a remote region of the Himalaya Mountains, in what is today part of Pakistan. He observed how the yearly inundation of the Hunzas' fields by glacial melting remineralized the soil. The alternating swelling and contraction of the glacier ground the surface of the mountain underneath it to dust. This mineral dust fed the soil every year, resulting in abundant, healthy crops and fruit trees with unusually long life spans.

McCarrison's book *Studies in Deficiency Disease*,[3] published in 1921, demonstrated that the more minerals a soil contains, the higher the mineral, vitamin, and protein content in the plants grown in it. McCarrison's studies would influence many others in the health professions, including Dr. Weston A. Price, whose book *Nutrition and Physical Degeneration* presents an illuminating record of what happened to the health of indigenous peoples across the globe when they switched from their traditional diet to the modern "foods of commerce," i.e., devitalized, processed foods.[4]

McCarrison's work also influenced the work of Dr. Royal Lee, who developed his own theory of the endocrine-nutrition connection after he began keeping a notebook about nutrition and health as a teenager. By 1915, Dr. Lee was convinced, as McCarrison would confirm in 1921, that the endocrine system was indeed the first system to break down as a result of malnutrition. Sir McCarrison also served as J. I. Rodale's mentor in the launching of the latter's nutritional publishing empire.

The forces of heredity definitely tend to inflict upon unborn children the penalties of poor judgment and carelessness that their mothers and fathers exercised in selecting their food. These penalties accumulate, each generation paying a greater price in lost health. A race that fails to take notice of dietary problems soon dies out. Dr. Weston A. Price found in his travels and studies of primitive peoples that they had accumulated a remarkable folklore of nutritional information passed down from generation to generation. Now we can see that this is not so remarkable. The existence of the people he studies is actually dependent upon that folklore. Those families who failed to accurately transmit this information, to take the trouble to learn the necessary facts of life, dwindled into nothing. We think we are of higher intelligence, but are actually being subjected to that same test.

—Dr. Royal Lee

[3] *Studies in Deficiency Disease* is presently out of print and no longer in copyright; it is now in the public domain. Selene River Press offers it—at no charge—as a downloadable pdf in the Historical Archives section of its website at **seleneriverpress.com**.

[4] For more information about Dr. Price's book, see the Books section of the Appendix.

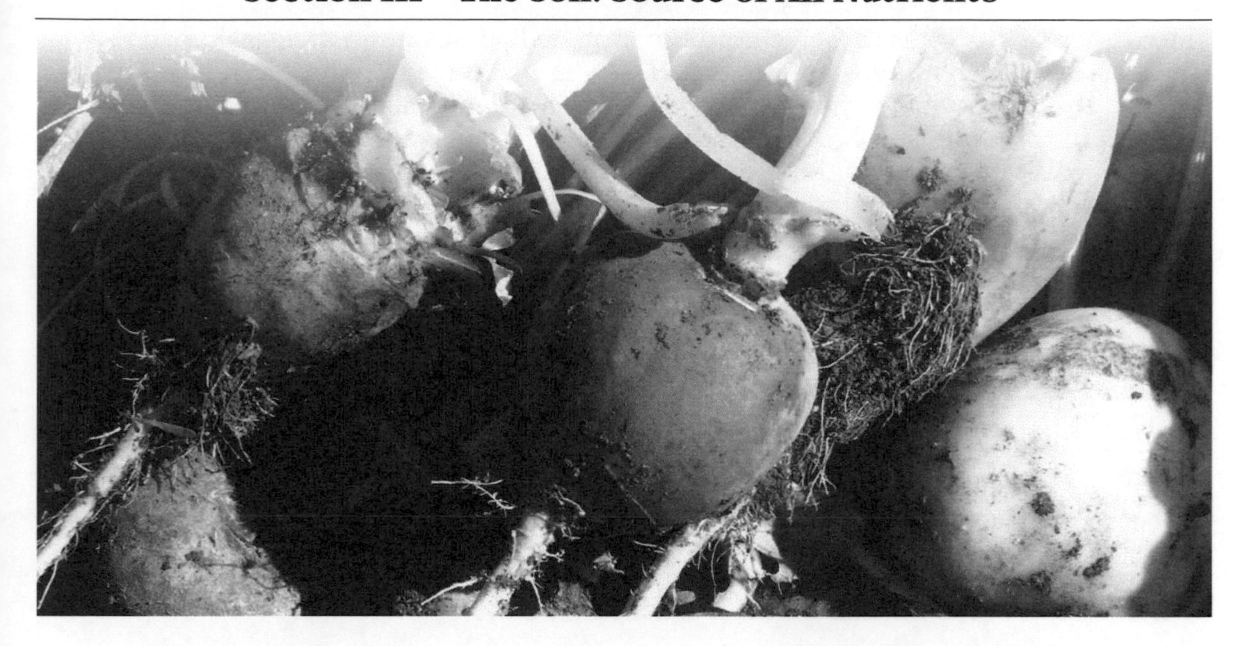

The modern farmer treats the plant; the true farmer treats the soil.
—Mark R. Anderson

A plant is only as healthy as the soil in which it grows. Plants do not manufacture minerals; they absorb them from the soil. Plants *do* manufacture vitamins, proteins, fats, and carbohydrates, but without minerals, the vitamins cannot function as catalysts. Mineral-deficient plants also lack both quality and quantity of proteins. *Only fertile, balanced soil yields healthy, nutritious plants, vegetables, and livestock.*

What Makes Soil Fertile?

Living **microbes** as well as over 32 elements known as **trace minerals** make soil fertile. These beneficial microorganisms feed on organic matter in the soil, breaking down complex substances into more-basic elements without which plants would starve.

Soil lacking beneficial microbes ceases to be a life-giving biomass because these microorganisms alone facilitate the cycling of carbon, calcium, phosphorus, sulfur, and other minerals essential to the health of plants and animals. Microbes such as nitrogen-fixing bacteria stimulate the growth of plants, while others such as fungi assist the transference of minerals from the soil into plant roots.

It has been estimated that 1,000 square feet of healthy topsoil contains up to 12,000 pounds of beneficial microbes. Thus, you can see why agricultural chemicals are so counterproductive in the long run: they kill soil microbes. Without the living bridge of microorganisms to connect the soil to the plant, soil becomes infertile.[5]

[5] See *Empty Harvest*, by Mark R. Anderson, in the Books section of the Appendix.

Trace Minerals: Organic versus Inorganic

Trace minerals—such as copper, chromium, iron, iodine, selenium, magnesium, and zinc—occur in such minute quantities that they're measured in parts per million. Yet they are absolutely vital at these amounts for the health of plants and animals. Plants deficient in trace minerals become stressed, unhealthy, and susceptible to disease. And trace minerals are critical to the complex electrochemical mechanism that is your body. Without them, vitamins fail to function.

While trace minerals occur in the soil and in plants and animals, the form in which they occur differs. In the soil, trace minerals are inorganically bound, while in plants and animals, they're organically bound. The inorganic minerals in soil bind with plant proteins in a process called chelation. During their life cycle, plants transform inorganic soil minerals into organically bound minerals that your body can use.

To further illustrate this point, consider kale and oyster shells. Both are sources of calcium. Which would you rather have with dinner? Even if you chose oyster shells, your body would know the difference and be unable to use this inorganic form of calcium. Yet many manufacturers of nutritional supplements use oyster-shell calcium in their products. In providing an inorganic mineral over an organic one, these manufacturers fail to offer a form of the mineral that will benefit the body.

Starve the Soil, Starve Ourselves

Nothing on Earth works as efficiently as plants to manufacture the sustenance of life for all other life forms. From the oxygen we breathe to the vitamins, minerals, and proteins of our cells, the soil-born plant is our ultimate link to life on this planet. It is no wonder we call industrial factories "plants"! Nor is it difficult to see how nutritional deficiencies begin in the soil.

When a person or animal digests plant protein, they absorb minerals. But for a plant to deliver its mineral payload, it requires a rich supply of trace minerals from the soil. To transform the mineral kingdom into the human and animal kingdoms, the vegetable kingdom must have high-quality soil, rich in microbes and nutrients from organic matter.

Today, however, most commercial farmers use methods that sterilize and deplete the soil, producing weak and deficient plants. They then apply toxic chemicals to keep these sickly plants alive and force them to produce deficient fruits and vegetables. (It's hard work trying to ward off Nature's intelligent effort to destroy inferior food!) Harmful levels of chemicals such as pesticides and herbicides also diminish the bio-availability of nutrients and can lead to disease.

Chemically treated, chemically fed, and chemically contaminated foods are the harvest of starving soil. Sadly, rather than entering into a partnership with Nature, most farmers today have unknowingly declared war against it.

The Price of Agricultural Pollution

In 1853, Justice Von Liebig wrote his landmark book *Agricultural Chemistry*, forging the marriage of farming and the chemical industry. Less than 50 years later, scientists and doctors began to speak out against the poisoning of the food supply caused by the application of synthetic chemicals to the land. But it was Rachael Carson in 1962, with her book *Silent Spring*, who captured the awareness of popular culture with the visual imagery of a spring without birds. *Today, agricultural pollution accounts for more pollution worldwide than all other forms of pollution combined.* Rain washes these toxins into our streams, rivers, oceans, and underground aquifers.

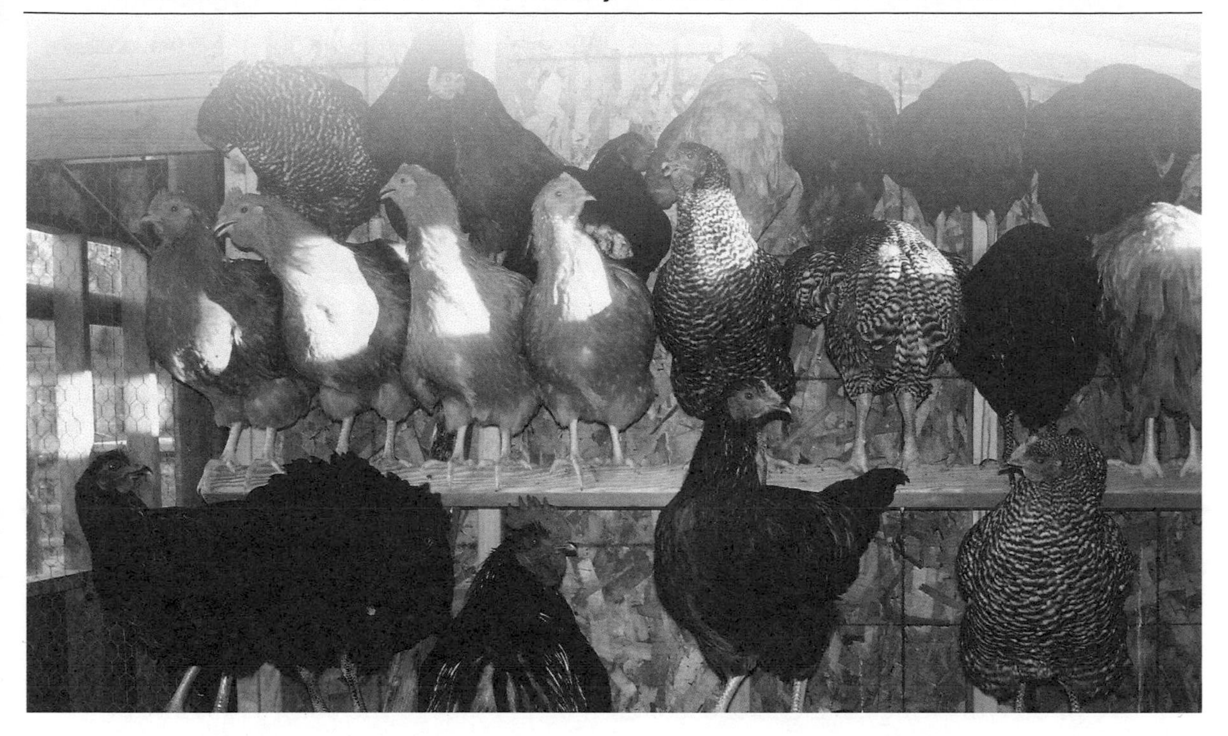

The quest for superior nutrition has never been easy. Historically, it demanded a deft combination of art and instinct, whether it was the cunning of the hunter or the wisdom of the cook. Today, finding stuff to eat is easy; all we have to do is go to the grocery store! But with this convenience has come a price: the loss of our fundamental ability to recognize nutritious food. To regain our understanding of superior nutrition, we must right some tragic misconceptions about the food we eat, shown in the list below.

The Seven Deadly Fallacies of the Western Diet

1. Chlorinated or fluoridated water is safe to drink.
2. Grains that are processed, refined, and then fortified with a few synthetic vitamins build a strong body.
3. Animal and dairy fats are dangerous to your heart, while refined vegetable oils, hydrogenated oils, and oleo products such as margarine are healthful.
4. Pasteurized dairy is a nutritious source of minerals, vitamins, and protein.
5. Refined sugar is harmless.
6. Vegetables and fruits grown on chemically treated soil are safe and healthy to eat.
7. Animals raised in feed lots and supplemented with hormones and antibiotics are a safe, healthy food source.

Surprised by the list? Here are some facts regarding the Seven Deadly Fallacies—facts we must all be aware of to regain an ability to recognize superior nutrition.

WATER

Water does much more than quench our thirst. In fact, it is one of the most important factors in maintaining equilibrium of the various body systems. Of course it is hydrating, but it is also essential for cleansing, lubricating, transporting nutrients, and regulating temperature. Would it surprise you to know water is also a source of nutrients? In its natural, unrefined state, it provides essential minerals, including trace minerals.

Just as with food, quality matters when it comes to water. Common water poisons include the additives chlorine, fluoride, and various water softeners, as well as toxic products of agricultural runoff, such as nitrates and nitrites. How much of these in our water is too much? As Dr. Lee said, "*Any* poison added to food or drink is too much. Like emery powder in a gear box, the damage is proportional to the amount and shortens life accordingly."

Chlorine—an oxidizing chemical bleach—is one of the most toxic substances on Earth. Along with killing dangerous bacteria in water, it can also destroy beneficial bacteria that live in our intestines. Beneficial bacterial flora are part of the body's first line of defense against ingested pathogens, denying harmful bacteria and fungi the opportunity to flourish within the GI tract and poison the body. Beneficial bacteria also help further break down our food for absorption. Without this aid, the body becomes starved of nutrients needed for growth, repair, and defense. The symptoms of such deprivation make up a long and painful list.

If you are not yet suspicious of chemical additives in drinking water, consider this: If you buy fish for a freshwater aquarium, you will have to dechlorinate the water, or the first thing your fish will do is...die! You must replace some of the bacteria that the chlorine has destroyed. Such naturally occurring bacteria in water, known as pyrogens, stimulate our immune system, as noted by Dr. Lee in a 1958 article in *Let's Live Magazine*:[6]

> Good water is water that has been filtered through the ground to reach the well or spring and has thereby accumulated a load of antigens. These antigens are otherwise known to science as "pyrogens," since they cause fever if injected into the bloodstream. They are the residue of disease-producing bacteria, and by drinking them we develop an immunity to the germ or virus that put them into the water. In foreign countries, where polio is relatively nonexistent as a known disease, the bloodstream of the children has been found [to be] loaded with antibodies to polio, which prevented them from contracting the disease. These children were immunized the natural way, not by a shot of Salk vaccine. It is very probable that their diet of unrefined natural foods that promptly supplies the necessary factors to make antibodies was responsible for their freedom from polio.

---

[6] See "Ideal Drinking Water," by Dr. Royal Lee, in the Articles: Water section of the Appendix.

Often, we dismiss an earlier theory as being unsupported by modern research, only to have science affirm the old idea. For instance, the following is an excerpt from a newspaper report on a study appearing in the scientific journal *Cell*:[7]

> Scientists at The Scripps Research Institute in La Jolla, Calif., said they were able to boost the supply of critical T-cells and curtail development of insulin-dependent diabetes in mice genetically cued to develop the autoimmune disease. The team, led by immunologist Nora Sarvetnick, reported a surge in the T-cell count when the mice were challenged with a mixture of bacterial cell-wall components. "Autoimmunity has been considered a condition of too much stimulation," Sarvetnick said. "What we are seeing is that it is a condition of too little stimulation."
>
> Sarvetnick and her team said their theory would explain why childhood bacterial infections decrease the risk for developing autoimmune diseases like Type 1 diabetes, rheumatoid arthritis, lupus and even asthma, and why incidence of these diseases has been on the rise in less-germ-tolerant, developed countries during the past 50 years compared to less-developed nations. "The cleaner everyone is, the less stimulation their immune system gets," Sarvetnick said. "Their immune system tends to be incomplete."

Clearly, the immune-building quality of unrefined water deserves more research.

Another common additive to drinking water is fluoride. Fluoride is medically categorized as a protoplasmic poison, which is why it is used to kill rodents. Numerous studies establish the toxicity of fluoride as well as its unfounded use for dental health. For more information on fluoride toxicity, as well as the effects of drinking water contaminated with pesticides and herbicides, see the Water Health section of the Appendix.

The use of water softeners is another way of turning healthy water into a refined non-nutrient. Water softeners work by demineralizing—particularly decalcifying—water through the use of salt. The mineral calcium bicarbonate, which makes water "hard," is one of the critical nutrients provided by unrefined water. Calcium bicarbonate is the most easily assimilated form of calcium for humans; it builds bone by combining with organically bound phosphorus in foods and lecithins in natural fats.

Unique forms of minerals and immune-stimulating bacteria make natural, unrefined water more than just a thirst quencher. ***Unrefined water is a food***. The only good thing about distilled water, on the other hand, is that it's wet. Distilled, deionized, and demineralized waters are stripped of their nutrients and in fact can even rob us of ours.

If you do not have a source of clean well or spring water running through your tap, then research the right water-purification system to remove pollutants from your water. Water-purification systems should be tailored to the specific water problems in your location. Local water districts, at your request, will send you an analysis of your water.[8]

---

[7] "Driven to Autoimmunity: The NOD Mouse," *Cell*, April 2004.

[8] See the Water Health section of the Appendix for more information on water purification.

GRAINS

Whole grains that have been properly grown and prepared will add high-quality vitamins, minerals, proteins, and fiber to your diet. Unfortunately, most commercial grains are anything but properly grown and prepared. As astonishing as it may be, grains that have first been grown on depleted soil, fed chemical fertilizers, and sprayed with toxic herbicides and pesticides are then stripped of the few nutrients they do have for shipping and preserving purposes!

For instance, commercial refinement of whole wheat berries removes the berries' bran (outer cover) and germ (inner core). This might be a good idea were it not for the fact that most of the nutritional value of wheat is contained in the bran and the germ. Each contains fiber, vitamins B and E, and minerals (the germ being more nutritionally dense). The remains are what we call "flour," which consists primarily of pure starch, i.e., carbohydrates. While flour does contain some minerals, the body can't absorb them without the nutrients in the bran and the germ. And what happens to the precious bran and germ? They're fed to animals, because farmers know they produce strong, healthy stock!

Freshly milled grains contain fats and oils that are as perishable as any other raw food, if not more so. They're like an apple, which turns brown as soon as it is sliced open. Oxidation is the culprit here. It turns the apple brown and causes the flour's oils to go rancid. (An experienced miller can tell how many hours ago flour was ground just by tasting it!) To overcome this inconvenience, commercial processors use chlorine-derived bleaches to strip the remaining oils. This process preserves the flour but leaves toxic chemical residues in every bite. Then, to try to compensate for the loss of all the natural nutrients in the wheat, a few synthetic chemical "vitamins" are sprayed into the flour.

Dead food does not spoil. This is why commercially produced flour will last for months in your cupboard. Sadly, instead of finding ways to keep people fed properly, food processors see the very beauty of living food as an inconvenience. Nevertheless, the fact remains that a living body needs living food—the only source of nourishment that builds living cells and living tissue. How, then, can we justify the processing of living food into dead substances that rob us of our health?

Fortunately, the marketplace has responded to the need for nutritious food. Whole grains that have been organically grown on chemical-free soil are now available in most health food stores. These include wheat, brown rice, millet, rye, oats, buckwheat, yellow and blue corn, spelt, amaranth, and quinoa. With a good home flour mill, you can mill such grains immediately before baking or cooking, which is the only true way to avoid oxidation and guarantee freshness.[9] (Flours should be used within 20 minutes of being ground to ensure freshness.)

In addition to grinding fresh flour, there are other ways of accessing the nutrition of whole grains—soaking, sprouting, and fermenting. Sally Fallon explains in her book *Nourishing Traditions*:[10]

---

[9] For more information on home flour mills, see the Flour Mills section of the Appendix.

[10] See the Books section of the Appendix.

We recommend the use of a variety of whole grains but with an important caveat. Phosphorus in the bran of whole grains is tied up in a substance called phytic acid. Phytic acid combines with iron, calcium, magnesium, copper and zinc in the intestinal tract, blocking their absorption. Whole grains also contain enzyme inhibitors that can interfere with digestion. Traditional societies usually soak or ferment their grains before eating them, processes that neutralize phytates and enzyme inhibitors and, in effect, predigest grains so that all their nutrients are more available. Sprouting, overnight soaking and old-fashioned sour leavening can accomplish this important pre-digestion in our own kitchens. *Many people who are allergic to grains will tolerate them well when they are prepared according to these procedures.*

With the consumption of improperly prepared grains so high in America today, it is no surprise that digestive disorders such as gluten intolerance and leaky gut are so common. Our ancestors, in their nonindustrialized societies, had the wisdom to know that *grains must be prepared properly in order for us to digest them.*

Are Carbohydrates Necessary in the Diet?

Interestingly, the carbohydrate form of energy is not essential to a state of health because the body can make glucose for energy from healthy fats and proteins. This is a fact proven by Dr. Weston Price in his studies of indigenous people who lived in perfect health on only land animal and fish sources of fats and proteins. That said, a reasonably healthy person can also maintain balance by including unrefined complex carbohydrates such as grains, vegetables, and fruits in the diet.[11]

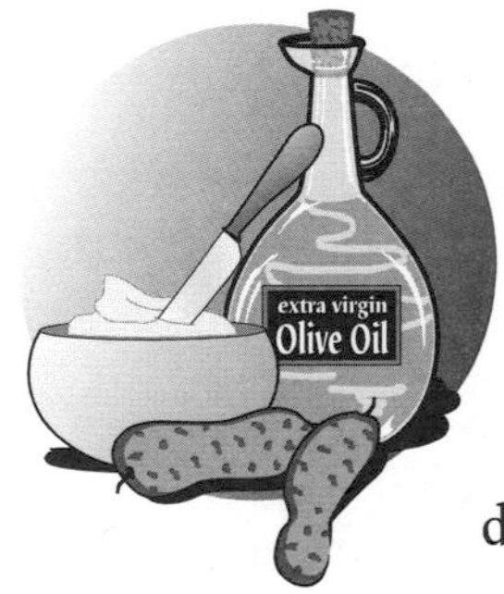

FATS AND OILS

Next time you're in the shower, ask yourself why your skin is water repellant. The answer is healthy skin is rich in natural oils, made from essential fatty acids you get in food. These oils also help skin retain moisture from the inside. If your skin is dry or you're bothered by skin or scalp conditions, you may be suffering from a deficiency of essential fatty acids.

Consumption of hydrogenated oils and oleo products such as margarine and processed cooking oils can aggravate skin problems. Why do manufacturers hydrogenate oil? Because, like the oils in freshly ground flour, the essential fatty acids in vegetable and seed oils go rancid in the presence of air. Hydrogenation preserves the oils and extends their shelf life by converting them chemically into something the human body has never seen before.

During hydrogenation, a seed or vegetable oil is first exposed to high temperatures and pressures in the presence of hydrogen gas and nickel. This breaks down the oil's molecules and reassembles them into a new form that is "saturated" with hydrogen.

[11] See *Nutrition and Physical Degeneration*, by Weston A. Price, in the Books section of the Appendix.

This new, synthetic substance has a higher melting point than the original oil, so it's solid at room temperature (think Crisco).

After the synthetic fat is refined, bleached, and deodorized, the product is finally reflavored and recolored for sale. The food manufacturer who buys the fake fat is happy because there's no spoilage in shipping, and the grocer is happy because the product with that fake fat lasts a long time on the shelf. Good for the manufacturer and the grocer—bad for your present and future health.

The human body does not benefit nutritionally from hydrogenated fats because the liver has difficulty converting them into forms it is designed to use. In fact, consumption of hydrogenated fats has been shown to contribute to vitamin deficiency, elevated blood cholesterol, and liver toxicity—conditions that can set the stage for blood, heart, gland, and skin disorders. This is why the U.S. Food and Drug Administration now requires food-processing companies to list the hydrogenated oil content on their labels rather than hiding it in the listing of total fats and why many wise restaurant owners have stopped using "trans fats," or partially hydrogenated oils, in their kitchen.

Because so many products are made with hydrogenated oils, it is important to read labels when you're at the store—especially at the health food store, since we tend to assume the products there must be healthful. Unfortunately, this is not the case. So be on the lookout for "hydrogenated" or "partially hydrogenated" oils in anything you buy.

So Which Fats and Oils Should You Eat?

The best way to get the fatty acids your body needs is by eating whole foods that naturally contain them. These include wild-caught fish, raw nuts and seeds, organic eggs, organically or naturally raised meats, organic butter (preferably unpasteurized), organ meats (especially liver) of clean animals, unpasteurized milk, avocados, olives, etc.

When it comes to fats and oils that have been separated from their source—that is, the stuff we cook with and put on salads—the picture is less clear. To understand, we must first look at how most seed, nut, and bean oils are processed.

To separate, or "extract," an oil from food, the food is either pressed in a mechanical device called an expeller or extracted using industrial solvents. While the former is far more preferable to the latter, it nonetheless has its shortcomings. The pressure created during expeller pressing a food hikes the temperature of the food's oil typically to 120°F, at which point oxygen in the air reacts with the oil at a rate about 100 times faster than at room temperature. We've already discussed the negative effects of oxidation on oils in freshly ground grains at room temperature. Multiply that rancidification by 100, and you start to get an idea of why virtually no commercial oils are truly fresh, even if they are "expeller pressed" and "unrefined," as oils processed in this manner are usually labeled.

For many oils, this is only the beginning. After extraction (whether by expeller or solvent), the oil goes through a number of high-heat chemical processes that not only strip the oil of its nutrients, including its essential fatty acids, but result in the creation of unnatural, toxic products such as peroxides, trans fatty acids, and mutagenic (gene-damaging) compounds. Thus, *regardless of how healthy an oil might seem, you'd be wise to steer clear of it if it says "refined" anywhere on the label.* Bear in mind also that processed foods sold in the natural food trade often contain solvent-extracted oils because they are cheaper for the manufacturer.

So expeller-pressed unrefined oils are not fresh, and refined oils are poisonous. What does that leave us for cooking with and putting on our salad? One of the best choices is **extra-virgin olive oil**, which is pressed at cool temperatures *and* unrefined—two things you're looking for in any vegetable oil. (Be warned, though, the term "cold pressed" by itself has no meaning. For instance, an oil that is expeller pressed and refined can be called cold pressed because no heat was applied during the extraction of the oil!) Other healthful choices for salads include unrefined, refrigerated **flax oil** and **hemp oil** (usually located in the supplement section). And, if you can find it, cold-pressed, unrefined sesame or walnut oil is a good option. Other than that, chances are that every cooking oil you see on the shelf—even at the "health" food store—has been altered by heating and/or refining.[12]

The best fats to cook with are natural and contain a fair amount of saturated fat, which is much more resistant to oxidation than are the unsaturated fats prevalent in plant oils. Such fats include organic **butter** (raw if you can get it), **virgin coconut oil**, and **virgin palm oil**. While many people worry that saturated fat may increase their risk of heart attack, in truth, scientific studies have consistently failed to show a link between saturated fat and cardiovascular disease. In fact, evidence suggests that the real dietary hazard behind heart disease is the overconsumption of refined carbohydrates and that, if anything, saturated fat decreases one's chances of having a heart attack![13]

Another reason people tend to avoid fat is the belief that it causes weight gain. Like the disproved notion that saturated fat causes heart disease, the idea that "fat makes you fat" is blatantly unsupported by scientific evidence. Again, the real culprit here appears to be overconsumption of refined carbohydrates. Both research and clinical observation show that most people who stop eating processed carbohydrates and start eating healthy, natural fats lose weight.

The failure to eat sufficient fat, on the other hand, can have tragic consequences. Consuming fresh, unrefined oils and natural fats is the only way the body can get the essential fatty acids—as well as the fat-soluble vitamins A, E, D, and K—that are so critical to human health.

---

[12] For more information on the damages of food oil processing, see *Fats That Heal, Fats That Kill*, by Udo Erasmus, in the Books section of the Appendix.

[13] For a comprehensive look at the research behind the fat/heart-disease hypothesis, see *Good Calories, Bad Calories*, by Gary Taubes, in the Books section of the Appendix.

Important Label Terms Regarding Seed and Vegetable Oils

Expeller Pressed: Oil was extracted from seed or vegetable using a mechanical press. Although no heat is applied in this process, the pressure created by the press results in the oil typically being heated to 120°F, at which point oxygen in the air reacts with the oil at a rate about 100 times faster than at room temperature, resulting in oxidative degradation (rancidification) of the oil.

Refined or Ultra Refined: Oil goes through a number of severe, high-heat chemical processes that strip it of nutrients and result in the creation of unnatural, toxic products such as peroxides, trans fatty acids, and gene-altering compounds.

Cold Pressed: Means no heat was *applied* during the extraction of the oil from the seed or vegetable. This does not mean the oil in the bottle was not heated, however. For instance, no heat is applied in expeller pressing, yet the oil is typically heated to 120°F because of the high pressure generated by the press. Also, *"cold-pressed" oil can still be refined, meaning it's exposed to all the high-heat processes of any refined oil.*

Unrefined: This is oil that has not been exposed to the high temperatures of refining processes. Unrefined oils are usually extracted at low temperatures and packaged to ensure minimal oxidation (to prevent rancidity) of the final product—that is, they are sold in dark containers and stored in the refrigerated section. Examples include flax oil, hemp oil, borage oil, evening primrose oil, EFA oil blends, etc. Extra-virgin olive, coconut, and palm oils are exceptions to this rule and can be found on the shelves alongside refined oils.

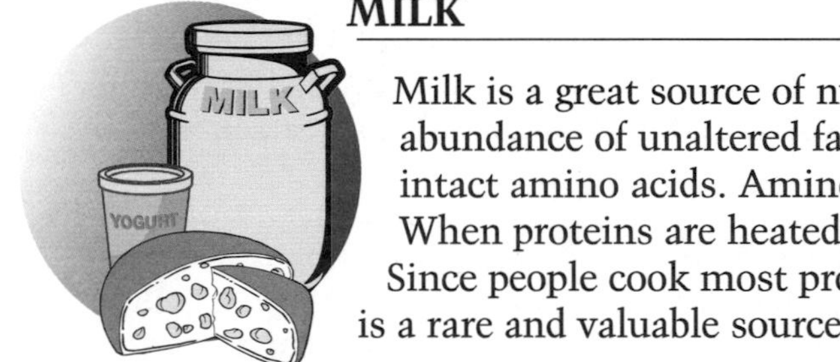

MILK

Milk is a great source of nutrition *if it is raw*. Raw milk provides an abundance of unaltered fats, minerals, vitamins, and importantly, intact amino acids. Amino acids are the building blocks of proteins. When proteins are heated, some of their amino acids are destroyed. Since people cook most protein-rich foods, certified grade-A raw milk is a rare and valuable source of complete, unaltered protein.[14]

Pasteurized milk, on the other hand, is a nonfood. A baby calf fed pasteurized milk, for instance, will die within two weeks. During pasteurization, milk's heat-sensitive amino acids are destroyed, leading to what Drs. Royal Lee and Francis Pottenger called "cooked foods diseases" such as arthritis and degenerative bone syndromes. Without raw milk's essential amino acids, the body's main connective tissue, collagen, degenerates and is broken down by the immune system.

Nor does pasteurized milk promote bone building. Contrary to what advertisers say about milk as a source of calcium, without the raw-milk enzyme phosphatase, which is destroyed by the heat of pasteurization, calcium cannot bond to bone! In fact, pasteurization kills all the living enzyme systems in milk. This makes pasteurized milk extremely difficult to digest and can lead to allergies and constipation.[15] Many people who have trouble digesting pasteurized milk experience no problems at all with raw milk.

---

[14] For more information about raw milk and how to obtain it in your state, see the Books, Online Resources, Foundations, and Food Sources sections of the Appendix.

[15] See Section VII, Nutrition and the Digestive System.

If Nature provides such a valuable food in raw milk, why then do we destroy its value through pasteurization? Pasteurization allows farmers to sell unsanitary milk to dairies, where it will be heat-sterilized; sterilization disguises the lack of cleanliness.

Pasteurized milk also undergoes homogenization, a process that breaks down the milk's fat molecules so that the cream content is no longer visible. High cream content indicates high-quality milk. Homogenization allows a producer to mix all grades of milk together, removing any incentive for the farmer to produce quality milk. It also encourages illegal practices such as combining outdated milk with fresh milk for sale.

Not only is raw milk a great source of nutrition in itself, but dairy products made from raw milk are excellent sources of nutrition as well. The aging and fermentation processes used in producing products such as cheese, kefir, and yogurt make the milk completely digestible. Fermented foods are also important sources of intestinal flora, aiding the body's strength of digestion and cleansing ability. In addition, as mentioned previously, raw butter is one of the best sources of fat available.

Unfortunately, raw milk is illegal in some states—not on nutritional grounds but for fear of contamination. This fear has been proven to be unfounded, as documented by the Weston A. Price Foundation at their website (www.westonaprice.org). It is well worth your effort to locate a source of raw milk in your area.

REFINED SUGAR

In 1910, the yearly consumption of refined (or "white") sugar in America was about 35 pounds per person. Today, the typical American consumes over 150 pounds per year. As sugar consumption has skyrocketed over the past century, so have the rates of degenerative diseases such as heart disease, obesity, stroke, cancer, and diabetes. This is hardly surprising. Countless studies and doctors' reports show refined sugar to be an anti-nutrient that can adversely alter energy metabolism and cause nutritional deficiencies.[16]

When our primitive ancestors ate sugar, which they did at a rate of *less than 1 pound per year*, it was in a natural form such as that found in fruit or a honeycomb. So while we should all be working to reduce the amount of sweets we eat, it's just as important to replace any refined sugar with natural, unrefined sweeteners.

Recommended natural sweeteners include raw, unrefined sugarcane (sold as Muscovado or Rapadura sugar), grade B or C maple syrup, raw honey, unsulfured blackstrap molasses, carob powder, and whole-herb stevia. Also, fresh fruit and unsulfured dried fruit are good snacks when you're craving something sweet. All these natural sources of sugar provide energy that burns slower and more evenly than refined sugar and do not cause the drastic imbalances in the body that refined sugars do. They also retain minerals such as iron, potassium, and phosphorous, which are lost during the refining process.

---

[16] See *Sugar Blues*, by William Dufty, in the Books section of the Appendix.

What about Agave?

In recent years, agave syrup has become a popular choice of sweetener. Just what is agave syrup, and should you be using it? The agave plant is a type of succulent that grows in the arid regions of Mexico and southwest U.S. To make agave syrup, sap is drained from the heart of the plant and then processed to concentrate it and transform its complex carbohydrates into simple sugars, mostly fructose. Since fructose has a low glycemic index, many proponents of agave tout it as a boon for diabetics and dieters alike. However, examining the reason for fructose's low glycemic index paints a far less favorable picture of this simple sugar.

The glycemic index is a measure of how quickly and powerfully a carbohydrate, usually in the form of glucose, hits the body's bloodstream. Unlike most other carbohydrates, fructose is not converted to glucose before entering the body but instead enters as is. And unlike glucose, fructose does not move into the main bloodstream for circulation (the reason for its low glycemic score) but instead passes directly to the liver, where most of it is immediately converted to triglycerides—the building blocks of fat and a major risk of heart disease. Fructose also blocks the metabolism and storage of blood glucose, causing the pancreas to secrete more insulin to process this glucose and, in turn, increasing cellular resistance to insulin's attempt to move the glucose into the cells. Thus, writes Gary Taubes in *Good Calories, Bad Calories*, "Given sufficient time, high-fructose diets can induce high insulin levels, high blood sugar, and insulin resistance, even though in the short term fructose has little effect on either blood sugar or insulin and so a very low glycemic index." For these reasons, many researchers believe overconsumption of sweeteners high in fructose, such as high-fructose corn syrup and agave syrup, is even more hazardous and weight-promoting than overconsumption of white sugar.

The percentage of fructose in agave syrup ranges from about 55 to 90 percent, depending on the plant source and the method of processing the plant's sap into syrup[17]. (White sugar, by comparison, is 50 percent fructose, while high-fructose corn syrup is 55 percent.) Sap processing methods vary from low-temperature vacuum evaporation combined with natural enzyme action to high-temperature methods involving synthetic chemicals. Unfortunately, at the time of publication of this book, virtually no information on these methods has been made public by the various agave processors. So, at best, agave syrup is a whole-food sweetener that has been altered only by the action of enzymes upon being heated—either above or below 120°F (the latter case qualifying the syrup as "raw"). At worst, it is a refined, chemically modified product that resembles high-fructose corn syrup in composition and method of production. As with any processed food, it is in your interest to call the manufacturer and find out exactly how the product it's selling is produced.

Refined sugars such as cane and beet sugars (i.e., white sugar), filtered maple syrup, and pasteurized honey contain almost none of the nutrients they did in their unrefined state. For example, sugarcane processing removes all the nutrients from the cane except sucrose, a simple carbohydrate that constitutes less than 1 percent of the whole sugarcane plant.

An interesting study conducted in the Philippines illustrates well the difference between natural and refined sugar. It is well known that refined-sugar consumption contributes to tooth decay. In the city of Manila, the population was observed to have a high consumption of refined sugar and, as expected, a high incidence of tooth decay. But on the sugar plantations outside the city, where the workers chewed raw sugarcane stalks daily instead of eating white sugar, tooth decay was rare. Why? The minerals and protective factors in raw cane juice help the body properly process the juice's sugars. Conversely,

[17] The percentage of fructose is based on a survey of agave syrup producers. Typically, agave syrup is 70 to 75 percent fructose.

sucrose—separated from the rest of the elements in sugarcane—stresses the body's ability to effectively handle and metabolize sugar.

When reading food labels, know the synonyms used to describe refined sugar: cane sugar, beet sugar, sucrose, glucose, corn syrup, turbinado sugar, and brown sugar (white sugar with molasses added).[18] Also beware of high-fructose corn syrup, a chemically modified form of corn syrup that just may be the worst of all the sweeteners because it combines the insulin-hiking effects of glucose with the fat-promoting and glucose-metabolism-blocking effects of fructose. And, of course, steer clear of artificial sweeteners, which are synthetic products entirely foreign to the human body.

Also avoid pasteurized honey. Companies that pasteurize their honey heat it to over 143°F, at which point its enzymes and other critical nutrients are destroyed. Other companies use heated centrifuges to extract their honey. While the temperature of these centrifuges remains below the pasteurization point, in some cases it exceeds the 100°F limit at which the living components in honey begin to be destroyed. Such honey may nevertheless be called "raw" on its label. Other raw honey is "cold packed" or processed at temperatures below 100°F and thus truly raw. Honey labeled "fine filtered" or "ultra-filtered" has been heated and is not considered raw.

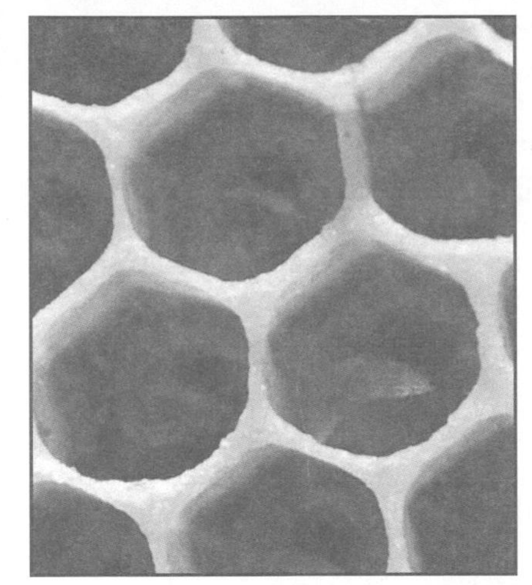

Raw honey can be solid or liquid, depending on the flower from which it was made and the temperature of its surroundings. (If the honey is liquid and its label says raw, you might want to call the manufacturer to make sure they have not heated it above 100°F.) However, regardless of whether it is solid or liquid, raw or pasteurized, all honey will crystallize over time at temperatures cooler than about 57°F. To de-crystallize the honey, place it in a glass container immersed in hot but not boiling water and stir.

Dr. Royal Lee on Real Honey

"When talking about honey, it's advisable to buy unpasteurized honey, because pasteurized honey is just as bad as pasteurized milk. It's a natural food, [so] even after it's pasteurized it won't decalcify your bones like [refined] sugar will, but it won't give you the vitamins. If you feed pasteurized honey to bees it will kill them.

"I have a letter from the Department of Agriculture to whom we wrote in and asked if it was safe to feed bees on cooked honey, the kind you buy in the store. It's all cooked, you know, to keep it from crystallizing in the jar. They said 'No, don't ever think of it because it will kill the bees.' So, that's the situation. We're eating food that's destroyed. Its food value is gone by simple-minded processing, processing that is totally unnecessary if we realized the consequences. It's just a convenience to the processor. He puts his honey on the grocery store shelf, and the customer objects to buying it if it's crystallized.

"Now let me give you a tip about crystallized honey. The only thing that crystallizes in honey is the glucose, natural glucose. If you take a jar of crystallized honey and turn it upside down over a plate with a couple

[18] For a more comprehensive list of refined-sugar synonyms, see *Food Fundamentals*, by Judith DeCava, in the Books section of the Appendix.

of supports across, to let the honey drain out and let it stand maybe a week (it takes a week before it quits dripping out), you will find that the glucose crystals that are left are absolutely repulsive to the sense of taste. You wouldn't think of eating it. Bees won't eat it. And if you dissolve that in water and feed it to your bees they will die. The valuable part of that honey is all in the fluid part that did not crystallize and which can be drained off and used. And you'll find that it is twice as sweet as the original honey. And another thing, the diabetic can use that drained off sweet and will find that he'll get no adverse affect on his blood sugar. So there are some interesting things about honey. Even honey, natural honey, has too much glucose and we'd be better off getting rid of it. And the bees are better off getting rid of it.

"If you want to accelerate this crystallization you could stir up the honey a bit and then put it away. In fact, if you put it in a food mixer and start stirring it, it will crystallize inside of twenty minutes. You'll get a honey butter. Well if you put that butter away in a jar, the crystals will grow bigger and then in a few weeks you can tip it upside down and drain off your honey. If the honey doesn't come out when you invert it, it's because you're trying to drain it off before the crystals have gotten big enough to allow the non-crystallized part to separate. But the part that does not crystallize is the valuable and healthful part. And the crystals themselves, after you've drained off the liquid, are nothing but pure glucose and are not suitable for food."

—Dr. Royal Lee, *Lectures of Dr. Royal Lee, Volume II*

VEGETABLES AND FRUITS

Back to Nature's factory—the plant. We've discussed how important it is for plants to be grown in healthy, microbe-rich soil, from which they can take up an abundance of nutrients and transform them from the inorganic to the organic state. In terms of human health, this means eat organically grown fruits and vegetables!

In his book *Empty Harvest*, Mark R. Anderson describes the connection between the soil and the human immune system, and documents how civilizations that once farmed according to this connection kept their people free of diseases that are now common in today's world.[19] Just as human malnutrition invites disease, the malnutrition we see in much of the soil today causes insect, fungal, and bacterial disease in plants.

The ability of a plant to survive without "drugs" such as fertilizers and pesticides is a sign of its robustness and health. Just because a conventionally grown carrot looks like a carrot doesn't mean it tastes like one or delivers the nourishment a carrot should. In fact, it is the nutrient content of a vegetable or fruit that gives it its flavor. When fruits and vegetables are grown in depleted soil, as most conventional produce is, they don't usually have the concentrated, complex flavors you get from plants grown in healthy, nutrient-dense soil. Is it any wonder why kids don't want to eat their vegetables?

Fortunately, organically grown fruits and vegetables are now widely available. Yet all the shopping in the best food markets cannot substitute for the experience of growing your own vegetables and fruits. Make yourself a small plot of dirt and plant some seeds. Even potted lettuce, tomatoes, and herbs will grow well in any sunny location and can be moved around easily. Beautiful, whole food—fresh and vibrant from the air, sun, and soil—is what it's all about.

[19] See *Empty Harvest* in the Books section of the Appendix.

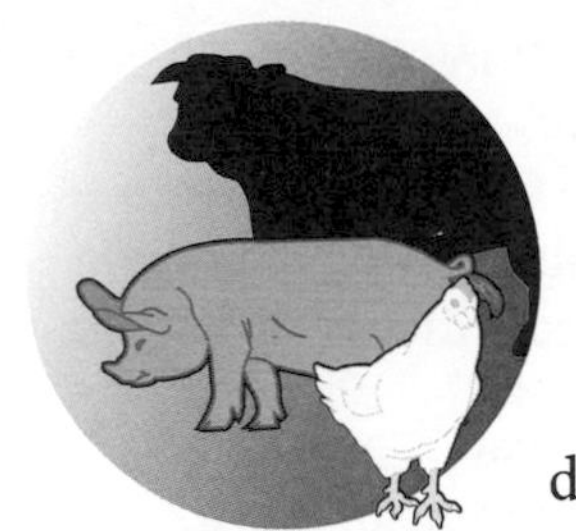

MEAT

Vegetarians often claim that animal products shorten life span, while some meat eaters wonder if a vegetarian diet can possibly be healthy. Arguments in favor of either can be made and supported.[20] In her book *Nourishing Traditions*, Sally Fallon makes the case for a diet rich in animal products:

> Russians from the Caucasus Mountains, an area famous for longevity, eat fatty meat and whole milk products frequently. Studies of Soviet Georgian populations show that those who have the most meat and fat in their diets live the longest. Inhabitants of Vilcabamba in Ecuador, known for their longevity, consume a variety of animal foods including whole milk and fatty pork. The long-lived people of Hunza consume animal protein in the form of high-fat goat milk products. On the other hand, the vegetarian inhabitants of southern India have one of the shortest life spans in the world.

The research represented in the previous quote is but a fraction of a large body of research demonstrating that animal meat and fat in the diet provides the highest quality and greatest concentration of nutrients necessary for human health. That said, however, bear in mind that our ancestors ate meat that was (1) only lightly cooked (preserving the integrity of its proteins), and (2) raised in the wild—or "free-range"—on soil, water, and land that was unpolluted by toxic chemicals. Also, when early peoples ate animals, they ate the glands, organs, and cartilage (gristle), which contain an even higher concentration of nutrients than the flesh.

The amount and quality of nutrients in such meat is hard to beat. But some people—perhaps because of the difficulty and expense of obtaining healthy meat, or because of poor digestion, or for philosophical reasons—opt for a vegetarian diet and have been successful in creating one that works for them. We must each discover and respect our own biochemical individuality.

As stated, our ancestors did not overcook their meat, which "denatures" the meat's proteins. Other processes that destroy proteins in food include overprocessing and hydrolyzing. Hydrolyzed soy protein, for example, is a common ingredient in many protein powders. Unfortunately, rather than using this substance as a high-quality protein, our body actually processes most of it as a sugar.

The central point is this: If you consume meat, it must be healthy meat. Know the source of the meat and how it was raised. When you invest in a computer or a car, you make it your business to know the manufacturer's reputation. So it must be with meat. Meat from animals raised organically or locally[21] is increasingly available in grocery stores, and many organic-meat producers are putting their names on their products and maintaining websites to inform customers of their philosophies and methods of animal husbandry.

Meat is another food that is worth raising yourself, even if it's just a few chickens or a goat. When you "get up close and personal" with the life that will nurture you and your family, eating is restored to the sacred act it was meant to be. For one thing, it would be much more difficult to knowingly apply toxic substances to the food you feed to your children.

---

[20] See "Food Fights, Part I and II," by Judith DeCava, in the Articles: Food section of the Appendix.

[21] Know the practices of the ranches you buy meat from. "Organic" means the animal was raised on organically grown feed and was not administered any synthetic chemicals during its life. "Natural" means only that no synthetics were added to the meat *after* the animal was killed.

We might cringe at the thought of eating an animal we've come to know. It makes us feel sad to kill a creature we've raised. And it should. It should make us feel many things, such as humble in the face of such ultimate sacrifice. If we close our eyes to these facts of life, we are protecting ourselves from feeling any connection to the animal. But to raise a creature for food is to experience deep respect and humility for the gift of life in all forms.

Granted, raising animals for meat might not be an option for you. Instead, you might want to consider raising chickens for eggs, or a cow for milk, bees for honey, or a fruit tree. In any case, raising your own food and knowing what you're putting into your family's bodies makes it easier to appreciate the need to keep the food free of toxins and rich in nutrients. But if raising food isn't an option, a great way to get more personal with plants and animals is to get involved in Community Supported Agriculture (CSA).[22] Or perhaps a local farmer or rancher would appreciate some volunteer help now and then. One of the quickest ways to check for a CSA farm where you live is to go to www.google.com and type in the following search query exactly as follows: "community supported agriculture" + [the name of your state].

Happy hunting!

Why Your Doctor Offers Nutritional Supplements

Now that we've considered each of the seven deadly fallacies of the Western Diet, we hope you can see why high-quality nutritional supplements are necessary. In an ideal world, clean water and healthy foods would be the norm. People wouldn't eat refined sugar or fake fat or cooked milk but would consume fresh food from plants grown on nutrient-dense soil, as well as untreated animals that ate such plants. Instead, just by eating the standard American diet, we are starving our bodies of the very nutrients that food is supposed to deliver. While better food choices will certainly put us on the path to superior nutrition, most of us require a jump start to begin regaining our balance. Potent, concentrated, whole-food supplements—made from healthy food grown on healthy soil—are that jump start.

[22] For more information about Community Supported Agriculture, see the Food Sources section of the Appendix.

Dr. Royal Lee on the Benefits of Real Salt

"We tend to have sodium deficiency when we do not include enough table salt in our diet. This is aggravated in hot weather when perspiration losses further deplete sodium reserves. Herbivorous animals need extra salt to compensate for the high potassium intake in vegetables, 'salt licks' being evidence of their need. Children deprived of salt have been known to crave soup (sodium oleate) because of its sodium content. Sodium compounds in any other form than sodium chloride—ordinary table salt—may be detrimental. This same sodium chloride (table salt) is now available in a natural form of sea salt at all health food stores, and is preferred to the pure product because it contains many naturally associated trace elements. However, one should obtain a low-heat processed sea salt, as heat-treated sea salt will not support life. For example, salt water fish cannot live in water to which heat-treated sea salt has been added, but can live in water with low-heat-processed sea salt. This is just one of the many unsuspected detrimental effects when heat processes are used. Sodium chloride is an essential constituent of the body fluids. We cannot eliminate water by osmotic transfers—we cannot perspire, our kidneys cannot eliminate waste materials and poisons—without the help of salt. Therefore, it is important that we use it in the best form. However, it must not be allowed to take the place of potassium which is the more important mineral from a physiological viewpoint.

"Include in your daily diet plenty of raw vegetables and, if possible, at least a glass of raw vegetable juice per day. Organic, low-heat processed sea salt should be the salt seasoning for your foods, used in amounts which are compatible with the taste and, for individuals ordinarily considered healthy, need not be restricted as to amount. Do not forget that the body cannot make something out of nothing and the human body needs sodium and potassium for its normal functioning."

—Dr. Royal Lee, *Let's Live Magazine*, 1958

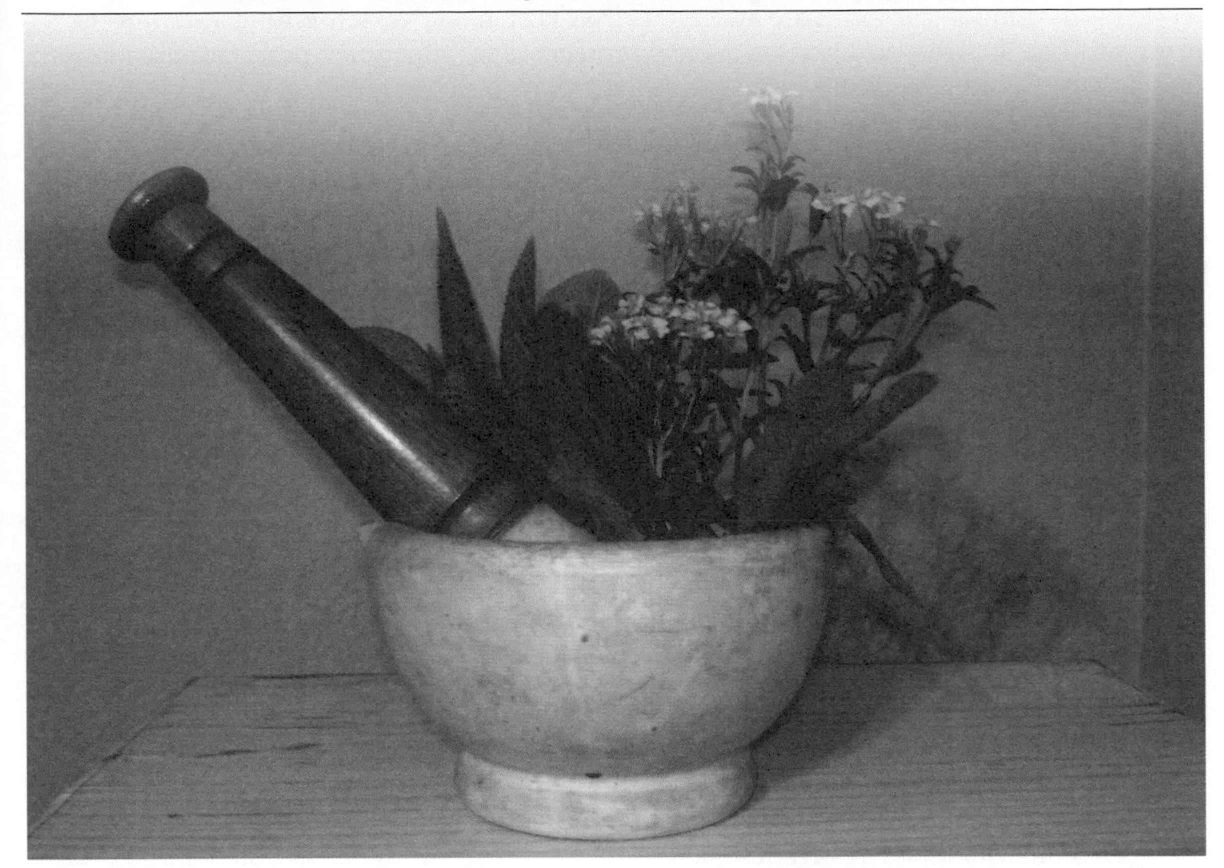

A good nutritional supplement program depends on many factors. In considering which supplements are right for you, your healthcare practitioner takes into account your diet, lifestyle, age, symptoms, illness and injury history, stress level, medications, handicaps, allergies, etc.

But perhaps the most important part of any supplement program is the supplements themselves. If a manufacturer's commitment to quality is not foremost, then there is no reason to swallow their pills. From the ground up, how a nutritional supplement is built will determine whether it will have the desired therapeutic effect or cause more problems in the long term.

Natural versus Synthetic

As we've said, living cells and living tissue require living food to thrive. So, just as the food we eat must be natural and unrefined, so must the supplements we take. Sadly, almost every supplement sold in health food stores is made from either synthetic chemicals or "isolated" (i.e., refined) food fractions.

For instance, according to government labeling laws, the legal definition of vitamin C is "ascorbic acid." Yet ascorbic acid is but a single, isolated portion of the whole vitamin C complex. In nature, vitamin C always appears as a combination of substances in addition to ascorbic acid that includes bioflavonoids, rutin, and organically bound copper in the form of the enzyme tyrosinase. Tyrosinase is the activating portion of the C complex, while bioflavonoids and rutin are synergists that keep blood vessels strong and prevent bruising. The ascorbic acid portion merely protects these functional parts from oxidation. It is as a peel is to a banana.

The early nutrition researchers knew that vitamins appear in food as intricate combinations of substances, which is why they called them "complexes." These natural complexes act collectively as coenzymes in the body, becoming part of the living cellular process. Synthetic vitamins, on the other hand, merely stimulate the body without becoming part of the cellular process. In essence, a synthetic or isolated vitamin has a pharmacological effect on the body—as illustrated by the body's rapid elimination of them via the urine—while food concentrates have a nutritional effect that naturally supports physiological processes. The body treats natural vitamin complexes not as waste products but as nutrients.

The Dangers of Megadosing

Vitamin C in the form of ascorbic acid is the most widely sold supplement in the world. Yet high dosages of ascorbic acid—an isolated chemical—can create a deficiency of its synergists in the body. In fact, prolonged use of high amounts of ascorbic acid, without the rest of the C complex, has been shown to cause mutation and degradation of DNA within the cell.[23]

Zinc is another example of the dangers of megadosing with synthetic nutrients. While a deficiency of zinc in the body will depress the immune system, too much zinc unaccompanied by the natural synergists found in food-complex zinc will upset the body's balance of copper, manganese, and iron. *Upsetting this balance also depresses the immune system*.

It's also well known that high doses of isolated, synthetic B vitamins can cause depletion of other B vitamins in the B complex and create health problems not just for the user but for his or her children as well. Dr. Lee explains: "I could write volumes on how synthetic vitamins like thiamine [vitamin B1] castrate the descendants of the victim who uses even as much as double the daily requirement." [24]

Natural Equals Balanced

The tendency for an isolated or synthetic nutrient to produce the same symptoms as a *deficiency* of that nutrient has been demonstrated repeatedly by scientific research.[25] This is because taking isolated nutrients creates imbalance in the body. Such imbalance may also result in *toxicity* of that nutrient. Both deficiency and toxicity are the result of upsetting the body's biochemistry by introducing a single nutrient without considering the cofactors necessary to metabolize that nutrient.

---

[23] *Annual Meeting of the American Society for Biochemistry and Molecular Biology,* Dr. Ian Blair, June 15, 2004; New York Times, Jane Brody, April 09, 1998; *Nature,* Dr. Ian Podmore, April, 1998.

[24] See *Lectures of Dr. Royal Lee, Vol. II,* in the Audio CDs section of the Appendix.

[25] For a detailed discussion of the effects of synthetic and isolated supplements, see Judith DeCava's *The Real Truth about Vitamins & Anti-Oxidants* in the Books section of the Appendix.

With food-concentrate supplements, on the other hand, balance is always maintained, allowing the body to fulfill its needs without creating deficiencies. Better yet, because of this completeness, whole-food supplements are highly effective at low dosages.

If most supplements on the shelves are synthetic, how can you make sure you're getting real, whole-food supplements? Fortunately, your health practitioner has made extensive study of supplement manufacturers and their techniques in order to offer you formulas that are made *entirely from raw food grown organically on balanced, chemical-free soil*, rather than heat-processed food isolates or synthetic chemicals.

Concentrating whole, chemical-free foods into supplements without breaking up nutrient complexes or destroying enzymes and synergistic factors requires some special processing techniques. These methods owe their existence largely to Dr. Royal Lee, who started developing such techniques back in the 1930s. (Now you know one of the reasons we mention Dr. Lee so often in this book!) The techniques developed by Dr. Lee help preserve the food's natural balance without breaking up its nutrient complexes or destroying enzymes and synergistic factors.[26]

Evaluating a Nutritional Supplement

If the planting, protecting, and shipping of whole foods require extreme care and effort, imagine how much more is required to protect and preserve the nutritional quality of a concentrated food supplement. In assessing any food-based supplement, here are some basic questions to consider:

- Does the label list the foods that are concentrated?
- Are the foods organically grown and in the peak of freshness when processed?
- Are low-temperature drying and extraction methods used? The best drying methods are vacuum dehydration (the most gentle) and slow air-drying (for low-moisture plants). Methods such as flash freezing damage cell structure because the expanding water inside the cells bursts the cell wall as it freezes. Any method involving heat, on the other hand, can denature proteins and destroy enzymes, vitamins, and other heat-sensitive components.

Evaluating a Nutritional Supplement Company

- Does the company have an internal laboratory for testing for impurities and toxins, or does it merely rely on letters of certification from third-party suppliers?
- Does the company allow visitors to inspect its operation and facilities, or does it just put out a fancy brochure that makes it appear to be professional? Don't be fooled by a company that won't allow visitors because it is protecting alleged "trade secrets." Any company that is proud of its food-supplement production wants people to come see what it does.
- Does the company conduct its own research and development, or does it rely only on the research of others?

---

[26] See About Dr. Royal Lee on p. 55.

- Is the company inspected? The facilities and methods of companies that make supplements from real foods must be inspected by the U.S. Department of Agriculture (and other government agencies). Check online for reports about the inspection results.
- Does the company conduct tests on every single batch of supplements for bacteria, fungi, pesticides, herbicides, environmental toxins (such as PCBs and mercury), rancidity, and impurities? This is a must!

Now that you know what to look for in a nutritional supplement, let's discuss some common questions about getting on a nutritional supplement program....

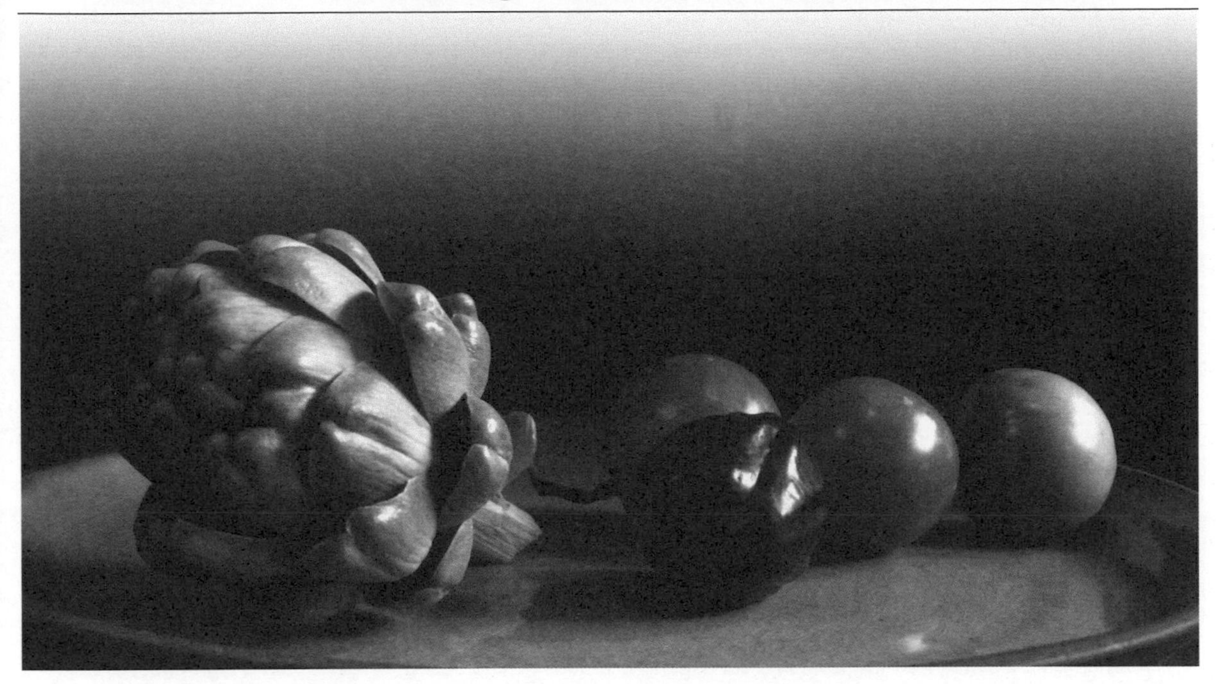

The nutritional supplement program that your healthcare practitioner recommends is customized to your body's particular needs, specifically supporting your return to health and preventing future illness. With that in mind, let's look at some common questions patients have when starting a nutritional supplement program.

Can Nutritional Supplements Cause Nutritional Deficiencies?

Yes! As we discussed in the last chapter, synthetic supplements and isolated food fractions create nutrient imbalances in the body, leading to possible deficiency or toxicity of the supplement taken or of cofactors that the body must use from its own reserves to process the isolated fraction. Whole-food concentrates, containing intact enzyme systems and made from foods that are organically grown on balanced, chemical-free soil, do not create such imbalances. Remember, when it comes to a supplement, balance is the key. Just as the human hand gets its dexterity from the relationship of the fingers to the thumb, a hand of all thumbs would be useless.

Are Nutritional Supplements Helpful During Pregnancy?

In every language, the first words spoken by a mother after delivery are, "Is my baby healthy?" The first words spoken by a woman upon learning she is pregnant should be, "Am I well nourished?" Half of all infant deaths in the United States are attributed to birth defects. Evidence shows such abnormalities are often caused by malnutrition during fetal development, at a critical time when nutrients are needed to form organs. Moreover, some defects in a developing fetus are revealed *only later in life*, making proper nutrition during pregnancy doubly important.

There is another reason for pregnant mothers to ensure that they are well nourished. One of the most unheralded findings of the early nutrition pioneers is that malnutrition during pregnancy not only affects the baby's health, but the health of later generations, as explained by Mark R. Anderson in the following excerpt.

What You Eat Affects Your Children—and Theirs!

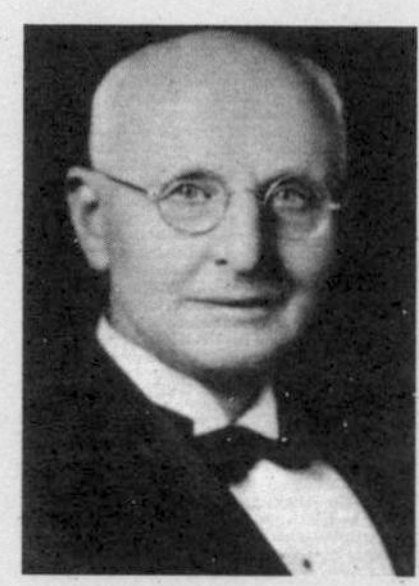
Dr. Weston A. Price.

"*Nutrition and Physical Degeneration*, published in 1939 by Dr. Weston A. Price, is an enduring classic with a message that puts the people of Earth on notice: Eat right, or destroy your progeny. During the 1920s and 1930s, Dr. and Mrs. Price traveled the globe to all habitable continents, photographing and recording the insidious effects of the modern diet on newly exposed indigenous people, their offspring, and their culture. Dr. Price, a superb field photographer, made a stunning visual record of the physical characteristics of native populations living on traditional diets and the subsequent altered features of their children as these family units came in contact with, and incorporated, modern adulterated foods. Irrespective of the setting—a naval base installation in the tropical South Pacific; a new trading post near the Arctic; roads built to connect previously remote alpine valleys; or encroachment of coastal cities into an arid expanse of isolated 'outback' (Australia)—the result of the contact and assimilation was always the same: the indigenous people were seduced into eating what Dr. Price referred to as the 'foods of commerce' (refined, processed, denatured, chemicalized non-foods). *Within a single generation, their freedom from chronic disease was lost and physical degeneration set in.* The next generation paid a high price, and it got worse with each subsequent generation: tooth decay, tuberculosis, physical deformities, arthritis, diabetes, diseases of the GI tract, infertility, cancer, and mental illness. Diseases, often lacking names or descriptions in the local language, soon became as common as they were in the modern 'civilized' population."

—Excerpted from "Prenatal Nutrition and Birth Defects," by Mark R. Anderson[27]

Because most people today eat a diet of the "foods of commerce," nutritional supplementation with whole-food concentrates is more necessary than ever for pregnant women.

Will Natural Supplements Interfere with Any Medication I'm Taking?

Nutritional supplements very rarely interfere with a medication. (Though medications often disrupt the function of nutrients!) Herbs tend to interfere more frequently. In any case, to avoid any possible conflicts, inform your healthcare practitioner of all medications or supplements you are taking.

Should I Continue to Take My Other Supplements after Starting a Supplement Program at This Office?

You should discuss all the supplements you are taking with your healthcare practitioner to see whether they can be harmoniously integrated with your current program.

Will I Experience Any Side Effects from Food Supplements?

The answer is yes—your improved health will be a side effect! In seriousness, food supplements can create reactions, but these are different from the side effects caused by drugs or synthetic supplements. Reactions to food supplements tend to reflect a

[27] See "Prenatal Nutrition and Birth Defects," by Mark R. Anderson, in the Articles: Pregnancy section of the Appendix.

dysfunction in the proper functioning of the body that can be very helpful in determining the root causes of that dysfunction. For example, if a natural food supplement such as wheat germ oil makes you belch or feel nauseated, this is valuable feedback on the digestive status of your gallbladder or liver. Now steps can be taken to improve your body's fat digestion rather than merely avoiding wheat germ oil, which is beneficial for healthy hair, skin, and nails, and is a rich source of vitamin E complex. Synthetic supplements, on the other hand, can cause adverse side effects. If you are taking a synthetic supplement and experience any such side effects, stop taking it at once and consult your healthcare practitioner.

Should Supplements Be Taken With or Without Food?

Good question! The answer is yes...and no. When to take a supplement depends on knowing the nature of the particular supplement and what it can achieve. Some herbs, for instance, work differently when taken on an empty stomach than when taken with food. One great advantage of receiving supplementation from a health practitioner is that he or she will know the best time to take any particular supplement.

Iron Supplements Give Me Constipation. How Can I Get Enough Iron?

The stomach prepares iron for absorption in an acid medium. So, if you are taking antacids and/or have poor gastric secretion function, you will have difficulty digesting iron. Also, most iron supplements contain an inorganic (nonfood) form of iron. Very little of this type of iron is absorbed, and what remains can cause black stool and/or constipation. Iron in a naturally chelated food form—and in a properly functioning stomach—is easily absorbed without causing constipation. Ask your health professional about the form of this important blood-building mineral that is right for you.

What about Supplements for Children?

The physical demands of growth can exhaust all but the best nutritional diets. Most children today are eating and drinking a chemical concoction of nutritionally empty "nonfoods," the likes of which no generation in history has consumed. The inadequacies and chemical contamination of our modern food supply make sound nutritional supplementation essential to the growth and development of children.

Do Nutritional Supplements Cure Specific Diseases?

No. Real, food-based supplements—like wholesome foods—support health rather than fight disease. They give the body the fuel and protective factors it needs for proper cellular repair, maintenance, and function. The supplements recommended by your healthcare practitioner will address your body's particular needs so that *it may heal itself* and be strengthened against future illness.

Paying Too Little or Too Much

There is hardly anything in the
world that some man cannot make a little worse
and sell a little cheaper and
the people who consider price only
are this man's lawful prey.
It's unwise to pay too little.
When you pay too much, you
lose a little money—that is all.
When you pay too little, you sometimes lose
everything because the thing you bought was
incapable of doing
the thing it was bought to do.
The common law of business balance
prohibits paying a little and getting a lot—
it cannot be done.
If you deal with the lowest bidder, it is well to add
something for the risk you run. And if you do
that, you will have enough to pay for something
better.

—John Ruskin,
Nineteenth-century English philosopher

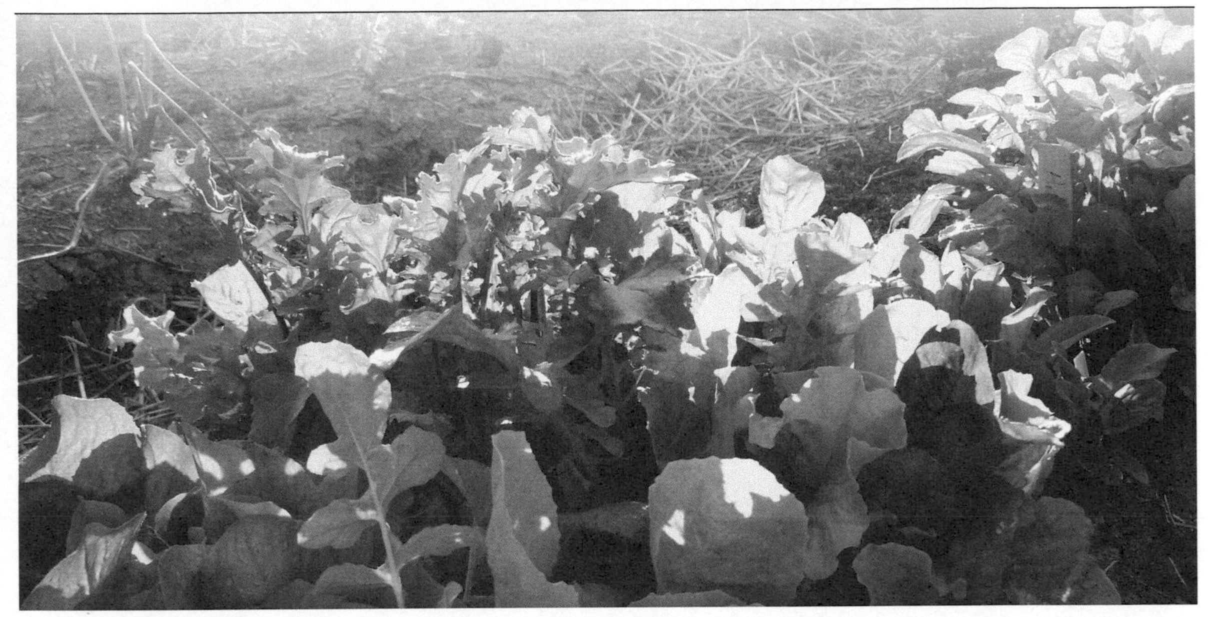

"You're not what you eat," nutritionists say, "You're what you digest." All the wholesome food and food-based supplements you can find won't do you any good if you're digestion is impaired or inefficient. That's because without properly digesting and absorbing the nutrients you take in, those nutrients can't get to where they're needed—your body's cells.

What is Digestion?

Digestion is the process by which gastric juices and enzymes break down foods into their essential components: vitamins, minerals, enzymes, amino acids, essential fatty acids, trace elements, and other organic complexes. These nutrients must then be absorbed across the GI tract into the body. Good digestion and absorption depend on many factors. Some of the most important are shown below.

Requirements for Good Digestion

- Thorough mastication (chewing your food)
- High enzyme content in food
- Proper hydrochloric acid and pepsin levels in the stomach
- Adequate production of digestive enzymes by the pancreas
- Healthy function of liver and gallbladder
- Proper balance of beneficial intestinal flora ("friendly" bacteria)
- Toned peristaltic action (rhythmic motion) of the intestinal tract
- Autonomic nervous system balance

The Importance of Stomach Acid

Of all the factors shown on the "good digestion" list, the most misunderstood—and usually the most important to remedy—is that of sufficient hydrochloric acid in the stomach. You cannot watch TV or open a magazine without seeing an advertisement for the most widely used drug in North America—antacids. These products are NOT digestive aids, as advertised, because *they do not aid digestion*. Instead they are indigestive relief! They merely counter the unpleasant symptoms of indigestion by neutralizing the organic acids that result from protein rotting in the stomach instead of being digested. This rotting process is what leads to gas, bloating, belching, and heartburn.

In the presence of sufficient stomach acid, proteins are digested properly and do not rot (thus no gas or heartburn). Unfortunately, people who produce too little stomach acid make things worse by taking antacids and neutralizing the little stomach acid they do have! This impairs their digestion even more. Nutrients such as calcium, iron, and vitamin B12, which require stomach acid for absorption into the body, are not assimilated. So a person who is taking antacids every day for relief from poor digestion runs the risk of developing anemia because of insufficient iron absorption, to mention one common scenario.

The popularity of antacids is evidence that many, many Americans are not producing adequate stomach acid and are suffering terrible digestion as a result of it. Beyond the immediate symptoms of gas and heartburn, it is well known that stomach acid deficiency leads to constipation and/or diarrhea, conditions that chronically afflict most North Americans. Proteins that are not broken down properly in the stomach can also ferment and putrefy in the intestinal tract, causing gas, bloating, toxicity and, quite often, allergies. Because the food is not sufficiently broken down upon entering the intestine, the pancreatic enzymes released there cannot break it down enough for complete digestion and assimilation.

Correcting Digestion

Eating whole, healthy food is a solid step toward righting your digestion. Such food is much easier to digest and assimilate than processed food—especially when prepared so that its enzyme systems are intact. You'll probably find that some of your digestive grief is remedied by eating more raw or lightly cooked foods, soaking grains, fermenting vegetables, souring milk, etc. Yet, if you've eaten a typical American diet for many years, chances are your digestion has been impaired to the point that some nutritional supplement therapy is still required.

It may be frustrating to find that a good diet may not solve your digestion woes. Fortunately, however, your healthcare practitioner is uniquely qualified to identify the right supplements to get your digestion on track. These will likely include hydrochloric acid tablets to aid your stomach as well as possibly digestive enzymes, liver/gallbladder aids, and even special blends of herbs and enzymes. He or she may also recommend a probiotic to improve the balance of "friendly" bacteria in your bowel. These beneficial bacterial help further break down food for absorption.

For most Americans, digestive therapy is a necessary first step in achieving the goal of superior nutrition. But there is another reason to get one's digestive system in order: The digestive tract is the first line of defense in keeping pathogens from entering the body. For instance, the stomach washes everything you eat or drink in its hydrochloric-acid bath, killing dangerous microbes such as bacteria, fungi, and parasites. (Another reason to make sure you have sufficient stomach acid!) In addition, friendly bacteria in the bowel also help keep potentially harmful yeasts and bacteria in check.

It may surprise you to learn that the digestive tract is such a big part of the body's immune system. As you will see, the digestive system is not the only surprise contributor to our body's defense.

Section VIII The Immune Alliance

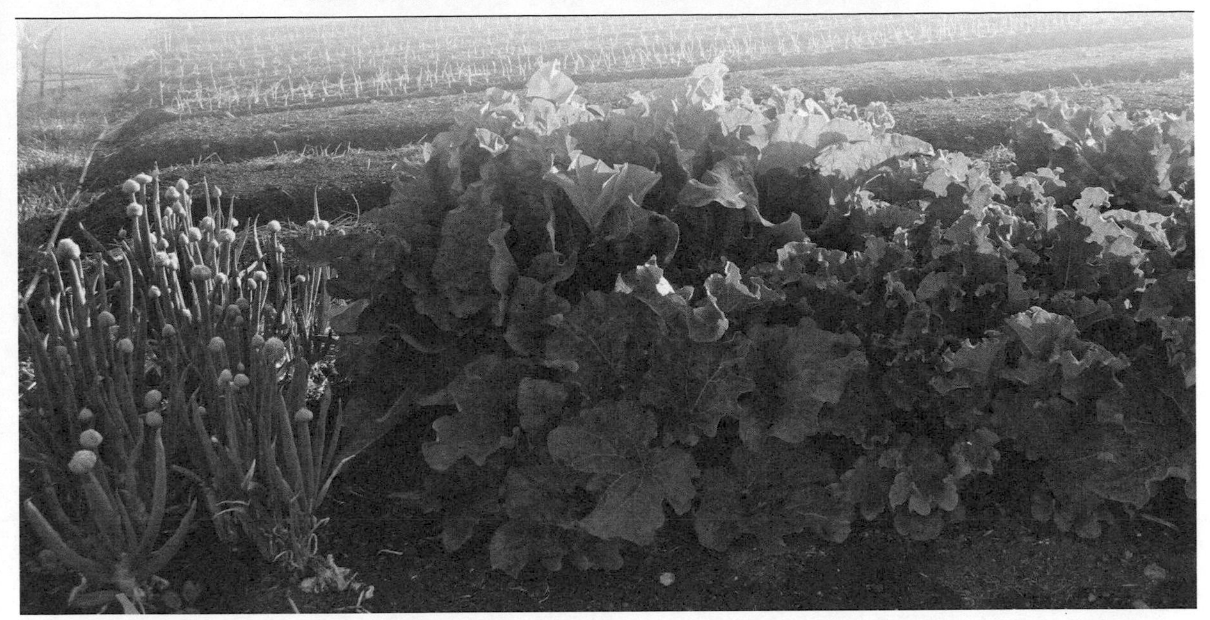

Although we constantly hear about the "immune system," in fact no such entity exists, at least in the way that we have a digestive system, endocrine system, or respiratory system. Rather, what is meant when we speak of the immune system is the defense reaction of an *alliance* of systems. In short, this alliance is designed to recognize anything that does not belong in the body, track it down, and eliminate it.

Think of how a city works. There is no single "Protection Department." Instead, an alliance of police, firefighters, rescue teams, ambulances, and hospitals cooperate to respond to various situations. Similarly, various systems and organs in the body cooperate to create immune reactions. This multidimensional network includes the liver, thymus gland, spleen, blood, skeletal system, digestive system, lymphatic organs, nervous system, and parts of the endocrine system. Together, this alliance expresses an intelligence, creativity, and self-preservation of unparalleled proportion.

The Allies

Although the immune alliance performs many functions, it is most notably responsible for identifying and getting rid of toxins, poisons, abnormal or foreign substances, dead tissues, and wastes from the body. The major players in the alliance, as well as their functions, are as follows:

- **Tonsils**: Collections of lymph tissue in the back of the throat that trap elements that participate in infection or inflammation.
- **Liver**: White blood cells known as leukocytes remove harmful toxins and abnormal particulates from the blood as it filters through the liver.
- **Thymus gland**: An endocrine gland that produces new white blood cells called T-lymphocytes (the "T" stands for thymus) that attack foreign substances (antigens) in the blood or tissues.

- **Spleen**: Filters out abnormal cells from the blood.
- **Lymph nodes**: Filter abnormal entities from lymph fluid and produce antibodies to eliminate bacteria, viruses, or other undesirable particulates.
- **Bone marrow**: The creation of all immune-related cells begins in the bone marrow, from which they are released into circulation for further development by organs such as the thymus gland.
- **Mucous membranes**: The body's "inner skin," which cover the respiratory, digestive, genital, and urinary tracts and prevents organisms such as allergens from entering through their barrier. They contain immunoglobulins (a type of antibody) to break down such organisms.
- **Skin**: Provides a barrier that prevents organisms and allergens from entering the body.
- **Intestinal flora and stomach acid**: Friendly bacteria and yeast in the GI tract deprive harmful organisms from establishing a living colony in the intestines. Hydrochloric acid in the stomach kills many ingested parasites and bacteria.

Nutrients Needed by the Immune Alliance

Tonsils	Liver	Thymus	Spleen	Lymphatics
Vitamin C Vitamin A Calcium	B vitamins Vitamins C and K Essential fatty acids Wheat germ oil Wheat germ	Vitamin C Vitamin A Copper Zinc	Chlorophyll (fat soluble) Iron Vitamin B12 Folic acid Vitamin K	Vitamin C Omega-3 fatty acids: • Flax seed oil • Fish oils • Cod liver oil

Bone Marrow	Skin	GI Flora	Stomach	Mucous Membranes
Folic acid Vitamin C Amino acids	Vitamins A and E Sea salt Amino acids Essential fatty acids Zinc	Acidophilus bacteria Bifidus bacteria Sour milk Yogurt Kefir Other fermented foods	Vitamin B1 Zinc	Vitamins A, C, and E Calcium Essential fatty acids

Clearly, strengthening the immune system is fundamental to strengthening the whole body. Your healthcare practitioner will determine which whole foods and whole-food supplements will best build and strengthen your immune alliance.

Beware False Profits: Navigating the Health Food Store

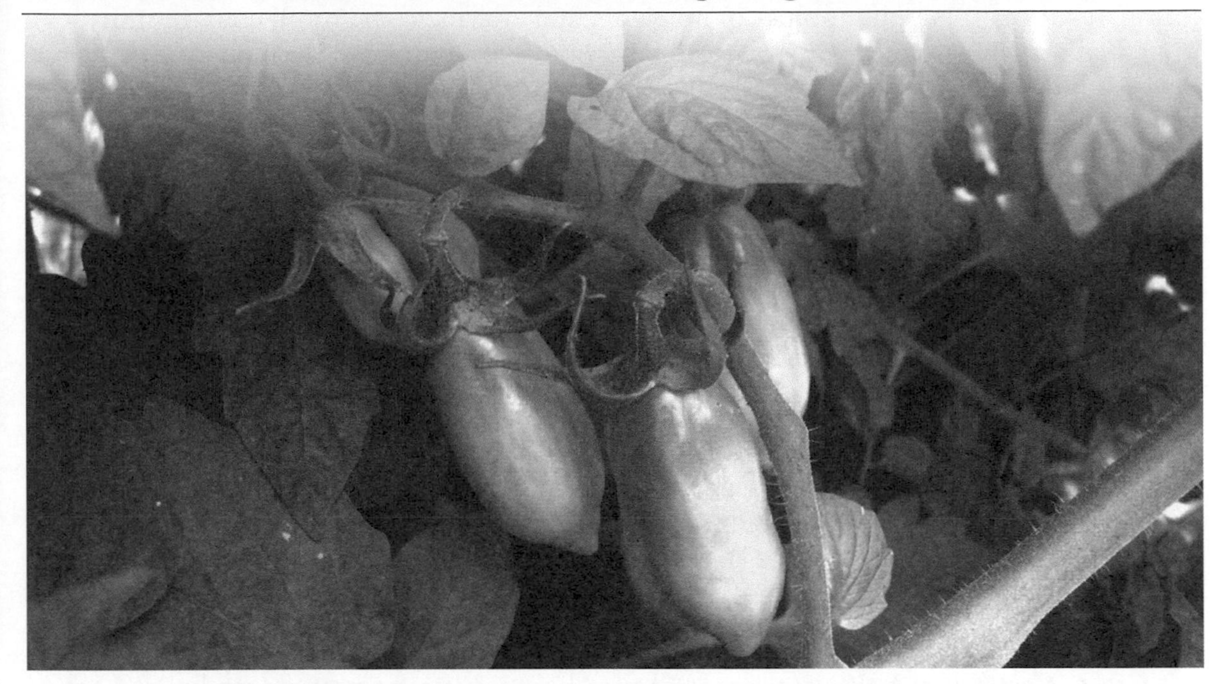

There probably hasn't been a civilization in history that did not have dietary beliefs about food and health. But to our knowledge, the health food store is a phenomenon unique to this current civilization and time. Unfortunately, the original vision of the health food store—to supply only honest, whole, fresh, organic, unadulterated foods—came and went with the 1960s. Today's "health" food stores do offer some of these foods, but thanks to clever marketing and grave misconceptions about nutrition, they also carry a *lot* of unhealthy food that is passed off as nutritious, including conventionally grown foods that are almost as adulterated as common supermarket brands.

For instance, bakery goods and deli foods in health food stores are often made with white sugar, white flour, and preservatives! These are not "whole" foods. And, one would think that a store truly dedicated to health would not carry *any* conventionally grown, pesticide/herbicide laden fruits and vegetables. Yet such produce is often more prevalent in the modern health food store than its organic counterpart. Even ultrapasteurized dairy products are commonplace in our so-called health food markets.

The reason for this is the main motive of today's health food stores is profit, not health. They offer what sells, not always what nourishes. Thus, it is our job—just as it was that of our ancestors—to learn to distinguish real food from counterfeit food at the health food store. It may seem unfortunate that we must be so wary at a place that claims to be dedicated to selling foods that promote health, but sadly, that's the way it is.

Counterfeit versus Real Food

So what exactly are "real" foods? Basically they are meat, fish, seeds, nuts, vegetables, fruits, grains, legumes, and dairy products in the forms our ancestors ate them—whole, unrefined, and grown on nutrient-rich soil without artificial chemicals. Counterfeit foods, on the other hand, are food products that (1) look like real foods but have been grown on depleted soil and treated with chemicals, (2) are processed into packaged or fast-food forms, resulting in significant loss of nutrients and enzymes, and/or (3) contain unfit ingredients such as refined sugar, altered fats, synthetic chemicals, hormones, artificial flavors and sweeteners, etc. As you will see, there are also foods that fall somewhere in between real and counterfeit, foods that have been compromised yet still may offer some benefits. While these foods are not ideal, they are at least a step up from completely counterfeit foods on your way to the superior nutrition of wholly unaltered foods.

The Health Food Store Checklist

In today's health food store your ability to discern real food from counterfeit is the key to securing superior nutrition for you and your family. Can you tell the difference between real and counterfeit food? Here are some of the important things to keep in mind when you shop at a health food store (or any other market).

✔ **Produce.** Amazingly, many health food stores stock conventionally grown produce in addition to organic. (If you wanted the former, you could go to your local supermarket and buy the same stuff at a lower price!) One way to make sure you are choosing organic is to check the sticker on the fruit or vegetable. If it begins with the number 9, it's organic. If it's a 4, then it's conventionally grown.

✔ **Meat.** Ask the butcher or person at the meat counter whether the meat was naturally raised, or better yet, organically raised. Was the beef grass fed or grain fed? Did the chickens get organic feed or genetically modified grains to eat?

✔ **Fish.** Buy only wild-caught fish. Farm-raised (or "aqua-farmed") fish is raised on antibiotics and nonorganic fish chow.

✔ **Oils**. Be absolutely sure to avoid any oil that says "refined" on its label. (Unfortunately this will be almost everything on the shelf except extra-virgin olive oil and virgin coconut oil.) This goes for mayonnaise as well, which is made mostly of oil.

✔ **Snack foods.** Believe it or not, many "health" food stores carry corn-syrup-laden soda, deep-fried chips, and cookies and other snacks made with hydrogenated oils and refined flour and sugar. Such foods offer copious calories while providing virtually no nutritional value—one of the frauds that drove people from conventional markets in the first place.

✔ **Dairy.** Avoid pasteurized milk! As we've discussed, the proteins and enzymes in milk are destroyed when heated to pasteurization temperatures. On the other hand, if you are lucky enough to live in a state where raw milk is commercially available, by all means buy it. Raw-milk cheeses are also a great option.[28] The dairy section is also where you'll find some of the "not quite counterfeit" foods mentioned earlier. Products such as organic cottage cheese, whole-fat plain yogurt, kefir, and cultured butter have the advantage of containing living cultures (i.e., "good" bacteria) and possibly some added enzymes, but they're made from pasteurized, denatured milk. While you're better off finding raw-milk versions of these products from local sources, they are a step in the right direction.

[28] Cheese made from raw milk must be aged at least 60 days to be sold in the U.S. Many imported cheeses qualify. At the time of publication of this book, however, the FDA was considering banning the sale of all cheeses made from raw milk. To find out about availability of raw cheese, visit **www.realmilk.com/where**.

- ✔ **Sweeteners.** Buy raw honey or unrefined maple syrup if you can find it. Avoid pasteurized honey or refined maple syrup.
- ✔ **Pasteurized juices.** Pass on these. Pasteurized juice offers nothing but simple carbohydrates (sugar) because all their nutrients and enzymes have been destroyed by pasteurization. Look for freshly squeezed juice, or better yet, eat the fruit whole. (You know, the way nature made it.)
- ✔ **Prepared and deli areas.** The foods in the prepared and deli food areas can be very enticing. But often they are made with conventional ingredients or laced with sugar-sweetened sauces. (If you wanted to eat dessert for lunch, you would dine in the bakery!) Even deli meats can be a source of hidden sugar. While some sugar is required for the beneficial fermentation process that works to cure many dried meats (and produces "good" bacteria), often sugar is added *after* the fermentation process, for flavor. As always, it pays to know how the food you buy has been prepared.
- ✔ **Baked goods.** Remember, flour is as perishable as a freshly cut apple; its oils go rancid very quickly after it is ground. Since health food store bakeries do not grind their own flour, this means the products they produce are made from stale, nutritionally compromised flour, even if it is whole-grain. In addition, almost all health food store bakeries use at least some refined, "enriched" wheat flour in their products, which is flour that has been stripped of its natural nutrients and spiked with synthetic vitamins.[29]
- ✔ **Breakfast cereals.** The processed breakfast cereals at the health food store may be made from organically grown grains, but even organic grains lose their nutritive value once they're processed into cereal. Moreover, such breakfast cereals are often loaded with sugar and refined grain flours, and some are even "fortified" with synthetic vitamins.
- ✔ **Fluoride.** Avoid all products with fluoride, including toothpaste. Adding a non-nutritive, toxic chemical such as fluoride to an otherwise natural product is blatantly unprincipled.
- ✔ **Supplements.** Almost all the supplements sold in health food stores are synthetic or fractionated, a fact that, as explained previously, is antithetical to the seminal concept of the health food store.
- ✔ **Don't believe what you hear.** The truth is, having read this book, you now know more about nutrition and food than just about anyone in a health food store. So when that man or woman at the smoothie counter wants to sell you a shake loaded with added sugar, you can simply say, "No, thanks." And when you hear an employee promoting something as healthful because it's "fat-free" or "made with healthy canola oil," you might let them know about the vital need for essential fats or the dangers of refined oils. Or you just might walk quietly by, content that you have the knowledge to know hype from health at the "health" food store.
- ✔ **Beware of health advice!** Health food store employees are not health practitioners and cannot be relied on for medical or health information. Healthcare practitioners study the latest research and findings and have the experience necessary to help others. It is far more safe and intelligent to find such a professional to guide you than to rely on the opinion of a health food store employee.

---

[29] Most health food stores use "unbleached" wheat flour. While this is good in that the flour has not been exposed to the toxic chemicals used in bleaching, the flour is still refined and therefore neither whole nor fresh. As with cultured dairy products made from pasteurized products, this is a step in the right direction but still does not qualify as superior nutrition.

While the Health Food Store Checklist provides an overview of assessing foods at the market, you can find much more information regarding this topic in the second book of the Quest for Superior Nutrition series, *Put Your Money Where Your Mouth Is! Guide to Healthy Food Shopping.*[30] By reading the guide and bringing your Health Food Store Checklist with you when you shop for food, you will not only make wise choices regarding your nutrition, you'll know how committed the store you're supporting is to upholding the principle of the original health food stores: to provide whole, unadulterated food to the general public as an alternative to broken, counterfeit food.

Alternatives to the Health Food Store

The free market is a great place for people to express creative ideas, make money, and contribute the gift of their unique dreams to society. But many of today's so-called health food stores are raking in the profits based on the pretense that they are selling healthy products. Regulation of these businesses in a futile attempt to police the integrity of business owners is not the solution. Such regulation has an antibiotic (anti-life) effect; it oppresses the creativity and freedom of those who do have integrity.

The history of the health food store industry is littered with pioneering health food stores and companies whose rugged independence was stifled by the huge conventional health food companies; they either had to close shop or sell themselves to a larger store. That's life in the free market. But the dominant companies have done us a great disservice by promoting cheaper products—sold at a premium—rather than expanding the market for real food. If health food stores had cultivated the raw dairy market, for instance, raw dairy products might be widely available today, and children would be growing up on one of nature's highest quality foods!

Part of the original impetus behind the creation of health food stores was to not just provide real food but to educate customers about it. Today the "education" you'll get in a health food store is a dangerous mix of marketing and misinformation. As a result, the line between real and counterfeit foods in the health food store has been blurred. That's why it's important when you're at the health food store to read labels, ask questions, write feedback in comment boxes, and call executives to tell them you want honest health food.

Or you may opt for something else. You may decide to dedicate some time and energy to finding places that sell *only* real, honest food, such as local farmers, community supported agriculture (CSA) farms and dairies, farm stands, specialty shops, and pioneering websites. The meals made of real foods from these sources will save you time and money in the long run. *Think less suffering, fewer medical bills, and no more sick days*.

If you find a vendor of real food that you want people to know about, please call or e-mail Selene River Press, and we will get the word out about them.[31] And, please call us if you find a source of raw, organic wheat germ that is nitrogen packed to prevent rancidity! We will surely reward you.

---

[30] See *Put Your Money Where Your Mouth Is!* in the Books section of the Appendix.

[31] Contact Selene River Press at 866-407-9323 or visit **www.seleneriverpress.com.**

If you're the owner or employee of a genuine health food store, let us know who you are, and we will tell the world about you! And thank you for sticking to your principles. Hopefully, the readers of this book now know just what a special service you are providing, and they will support your efforts in lieu of shopping at less-principled stores dedicated to profit over health.

If we teach children at a young age that by their eating habits they will determine the health of the next generation, they will learn responsibility in all areas of life. It might even be said that the lack of a sense of responsibility that characterizes so much of modern government and industry today is an outgrowth of the attitude that the way we eat has no bearing on the health of our children and grandchildren.

—Sally Fallon

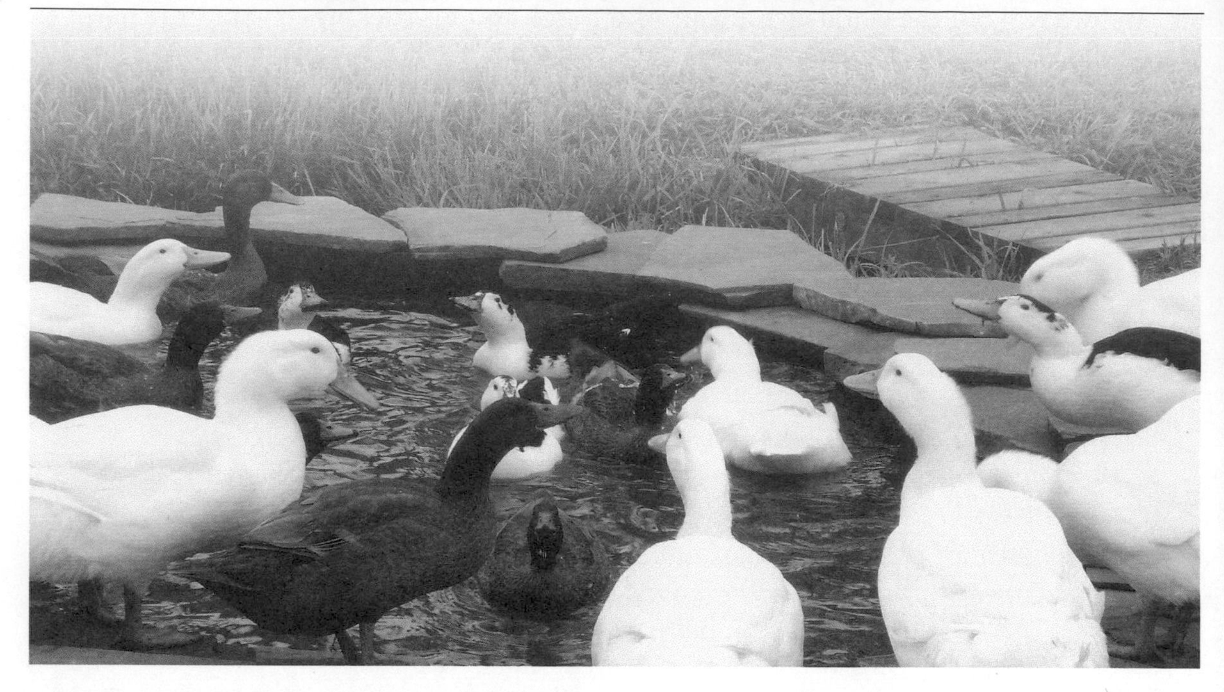

There is a lot of information about health out there. As you now know, having read this book, much of it is either misguided or simply incorrect. Supposed dramatic breakthroughs trumpeted in the popular press are often nothing more than hype. Fortunately, as you develop a wholesome lifestyle based on the principles you've learned, discerning what is true about nutrition and what is best for your body's needs will become easier. Professional assistance is a critical resource for information and guidance. Don't hesitate to seek the advice of your healthcare professional for information on how to accomplish your goals and where to find more knowledge and wisdom on nutrition and health. In addition, we highly recommend the following materials for further self-education and explanation of the fundamentals of nutrition addressed in this book.

Recommended Resources in the Quest for Superior Nutrition

Books

Don't Drink Your Milk! New Frightening Medical Facts about the World's Most Overrated Nutrient, by Frank A. Oski, MD. Available from various booksellers.

Empty Harvest: The Link Between the Soil and Our Immune System, by Dr. Bernard Jensen and Mark R. Anderson. Available from Selene River Press, **866-407-9323**, **www.seleneriverpress.com**, and various booksellers.

Fats That Heal, Fats That Kill, by Udo Erasmus. Available from Selene River Press, **866-407-9323**, **www.seleneriverpress.com**, and various booksellers.

Food Fundamentals, and all other books by Judith DeCava, MS, LNC. Available from Selene River Press, **866-407-9323**, **www.seleneriverpress.com**.

Good Calories, Bad Calories: Challenging the Conventional Wisdom on Diet, Weight Control, and Disease, by Gary Taubes. Available from Selene River Press, **866-407-9323**, **www.seleneriverpress.com**, and various booksellers.

Handbook to Health: With Menus and Recipes, by Vivian Rice and Edie Wogaman. Available from Selene River Press, **866-407-9323**, **www.seleneriverpress.com**.

A Hunza Trip: The Wheel of Health, by Dr. Bernard Jensen and G. T. Wrench, MD. See all books by Bernard Jensen, PhD, DC, published by Bernard Jensen International, **www.bernardjensen.org**.

Know Your Fats: The Complete Primer for Understanding the Nutrition of Fats, Oils and Cholesterol, by Mary G. Enig. (Mary Enig was the first person to speak out about the dangers of trans-fatty acids in the food supply in spite of industry blackballing.) Available from Selene River Press, **866-407-9323**, **www.seleneriverpress.com**, and various booksellers.

Lectures of Dr. Royal Lee, Volume I and II, compiled by Mark R. Anderson. (Volume II is a 32-CD box set; see section Audio CDs.) Available only through Selene River Press, **866-407-9323**, **www.seleneriverpress.com**.

Nourishing Traditions: The Cookbook that Challenges Politically Correct Nutrition and the Diet Dictocrats, by Sally Fallon, with Mary G. Enig. Available from New Trends Publishing, **877-707-1776**, **www.newtrendspublishing.com**, or Selene River Press, **866-407-9323**, **www.seleneriverpress.com**.

Nutrition and Physical Degeneration, by Dr. Weston Price. Available from The Price-Pottenger Foundation, **800-366-3748**, **www.ppnf.org**, or Selene River Press, **866-407-9323**, **www.seleneriverpress.com**.

Pottenger's Cats: A Study in Nutrition, by Francis M. Pottenger, MD. Available from Selene River Press, **866-407-9323**, **www.seleneriverpress.com**, and various booksellers.

Put Your Money Where Your Mouth Is! Guide to Healthy Food Shopping, by Stephanie Selene Anderson. Available from Selene River Press, **866-407-9323**, **www.seleneriverpress.com**, and various booksellers.

The Real Truth about Vitamins and Anti-Oxidants, by Judith DeCava, MS, LNC. Available from Selene River Press, **866-407-9323**, **www.seleneriverpress.com**.

Studies in Deficiency Disease, by Sir Major General William McCarrison, MD. Available as a free, downloadable pdf from the Historical Archives section of Selene River Press' website, **www.seleneriverpress.com**.

Sugar Blues, by William Dufty. Available from Selene River Press, **866-407-9323**, **www.seleneriverpress.com**, and various booksellers.

The Untold Story of Milk, Revised and Updated: The History, Politics and Science of Nature's Perfect Food: Raw Milk from Pasture-Fed Cows, by Ron Schmid, ND. Available from various booksellers.

See also all books on diet and health, including Sally Fallon's books, from New Trends Publishing, **877-707-1776**, **www.newtrendspublishing.com**.

Online Resources

www.bonanzle.com/booths/nicksnaturalnook, home of Nick's Natural Nook, is a fantastic marketplace for whole, natural products such as organic teas and starter kits to make your own yogurt and kefir.

www.mercola.com, headed by Dr. Joseph Mercola, offers reviews of the latest research into food and nutrition as well as book and product recommendations, and it has a great search function to find information among the site's vast database of health-related topics. You can also sign up for Dr. Mercola's free e-newsletter to get nutrition information delivered directly to your in-box.

www.realmilk.com is the website for Real Milk, a campaign started by Sally Fallon and the Weston A. Price Foundation to make fresh, raw milk available to the public. The site offers information about the benefits of raw milk as well as how you can obtain raw milk in your state.

www.jamieoliver.com/campaigns/jamies-food-revolution is home to popular TV chef Jamie Oliver's campaign to educate children and parents about real food. "This food revolution is about saving America's health by changing the way you eat," says Oliver. "Switching from processed to fresh food will not only make you feel better but it will add years to your life."

Periodicals

Acres USA: A Voice for Eco-Agriculture. Call **800-355-5313** or visit **www.acresusa.com**.

News and Views—on Nutritional Therapeutics, Vol.1–8, 1997–2004. A CD compilation of Judith DeCava's newsletter for health professionals. Available only from Selene River Press, **866-407-9323**, **www.seleneriverpress.com**.

Wise Traditions in Food, Farming and the Healing Arts. A publication of The Weston A. Price Foundation, edited by Sally Fallon. Available from The Weston A. Price Foundation, **202-363-4393**, **www.westonaprice.org**.

Articles

FOOD

"Food Fights, Part I and II," by Judith DeCava, CCN, LNC, *Nutrition News and Views—on Nutritional Therapeutics*, Vol. 5, No. 3, 2001. Available on CD-ROM from Selene River Press, **866-407-9323**, **www.seleneriverpress.com**.

PREGNANCY

"Prenatal Nutrition and Birth Defects," by Mark R. Anderson, *Whole Food Nutrition Journal*, Vol. 1, No. 2, 2001. Available free from the *Historical Archives* page of Selene River Press' website, **www.seleneriverpress.com**, or call **866-407-9323**.

VITAMIN A

"Vitamin A—Toxic or Terrific?" by Judith DeCava, *Nutrition News and Views—on Nutritional Therapeutics*, Vol. 8, No.4, 2004. CD-ROM collection available through Selene River Press at **866-407-9323** or **www.seleneriverpress.com**.

WATER

"Ideal Drinking Water," by Dr. Royal Lee, DDS, *Let's Live Magazine*. Available free from the Historical Archives section of Selene River Press' website, **www.seleneriverpress.com**, or call **866-407-9323**.

Audio CDs

Lectures of Dr. Royal Lee, Volume I and II, compiled by Mark R. Anderson. (Volume I is a book; see the Books section of this appendix.) Available only through Selene River Press, **866-407-9323**, **www.seleneriverpress.com**.

Foundations

THE WESTON A. PRICE FOUNDATION. In the foundation's own words:

> The [Weston A. Price] Foundation is dedicated to restoring nutrient-dense foods to the human diet through education, research and activism. It supports a number of movements that contribute to this objective, including accurate nutrition instruction, organic and biodynamic farming, pasture-feeding of livestock, community-supported farms, honest and informative labeling, prepared parenting and nurturing therapies. Specific goals include establishment of universal access to clean, certified raw milk and a ban on the use of soy formula for infants.

You can contact the foundation at **202-363-4393** or **www.westonaprice.org**.

REAL MILK, founded by Sally Fallon, is a campaign for real milk and a project of the Weston A. Price Foundation. "Back in the '20s," says Fallon, "Americans could buy fresh raw whole milk, real clabber and buttermilk, luscious naturally yellow butter, fresh farm cheeses and cream in various colors and thicknesses. Today's milk is accused of causing everything from allergies to heart disease to cancer, but when Americans could buy real milk, these diseases were rare. In fact, a supply of high quality dairy products was considered vital to American security and the economic well being of the nation. What's needed today is a return to humane, non-toxic, pasture-based dairying and small-scale traditional processing, in short...a campaign for real milk."

Find out more information about the Real Milk project at **www.realmilk.com**.

THE PRICE-POTTENGER NUTRITION FOUNDATION. In the foundation's own words:

"Through the dissemination of the ancestral wisdom practiced by pre-industrial societies, and through modern scientific validation of the principles of sound nutrition, the Price-Pottenger Nutrition Foundation (PPNF) provides guidance for the reversal of modern 'civilized' dietary trends that promote disease and physical & mental degeneration.

"The Foundation is dedicated to achieving the optimum expression of our human genetic potential and harmony with nature's laws through the right use of technology and the practical application of the principles of sound nutrition. PPNF provides accurate information on whole foods and proper preparation techniques, soil improvement, natural farming, pure water, non-toxic dentistry and holistic therapies in order to conquer disease; prevent birth defects; avoid personality disturbances & delinquency; enhance the environment; and enable all people to achieve long life and excellent health, now and into the 21st century.

"To [ensure that] healing professionals and the public would always have access to the critical nutritional discoveries of Dr. Price, the Foundation has a mandate to maintain in print his Nutrition and Physical Degeneration [since] it contains the documentation of his research."

You can contact the Price-Pottenger Nutrition Foundation at **800-366-3748** or **www.price-pottenger.org**.

Other Resources

SELENE RIVER PRESS, INC., Publisher and Distributor of Select Books on Health. Selene River Press provides a free self-education CD catalog, *The Selene River Press Collection: A Catalog of Self-Health Literacy*, and is dedicated to the publication and distribution of books, tools, and resources that support and guide lifelong learning in the art and science of health through nutrition. To order many of the self-education materials listed in this appendix, call Selene River Press for a free CD catalog at **866-407-9323, 970-461-4602**. Or, you can download the catalog at **www.seleneriverpress.com**.

Weston A. Price Foundation Shopping Guide: For Finding the Healthiest Foods in the Supermarkets and Health Food Stores, by Sally Fallon. The WAPF Shopping Guide is a handy pamphlet listing specific brands and contact information for many of the highest quality foods on the market. Available from the Weston A. Price Foundation, **202-363-4393**.

Water Health

FLUORIDE

Empty Harvest, by Dr. Bernard Jensen and Mark R. Anderson; ***Food Fundamentals*** and ***Conquering Cancer***, by Judith DeCava. See the Books section of this appendix for more information.

Fluoride Action Network is an international coalition working to end water fluoridation and alert the public to fluoride's health and environmental risks. Call **802-338-5577** or visit **www.fluoridealert.org**.

LOCAL WATER QUALITY

Check with your city for a copy of the "Consumer Confidence Report." Cities are required by law to make available this report about the contents of their water. All water testing done is public record, for the asking. For more information, call **202-564-3750** or visit **www.epa.gov/safewater/ccr/**.

PURIFICATION AND INFORMATION

Ozark Water Service & Air Services. A company dedicated to providing individuals information on water and air purity. Headed by Warren Clough, analytical chemist and water consultant. Call **800-835-8908** or **479-298-3483**, or visit **ozarkwaterandair.org**.

COD LIVER OIL

Blue Ice Pure Cod Liver Oil is a unique cod liver oil produced in Norway. The cod is seasonally fished and exclusively harvested from the icy blue Arctic Ocean, and the oil is molecularly distilled, all to ensure a premium quality, naturally high-vitamin cod liver oil. For more information or to order Blue Ice cod liver oils, call Green Pasture at **402-858-4818** or visit **www.greenpasture.org**.

COMMUNITY SUPPORTED AGRICULTURE (CSA) FARMS AND GARDENS

Community Supported Agriculture is a growing movement by which members of the community actively support farms in their area and receive nutritious, whole food in return. Typically, members of the farm pledge to cover some of the cost of the farm operation, for example, by buying a share in the farm's cow herd if it is a raw dairy farm. In return, the members receive some of the bounty of the farm, whether it be raw milk or organic produce, as well as the deep satisfaction of being part of local food production and supporting their local farmers. For more information about CSA farms and gardens, visit **www.usda.gov/afsic/pubs/csa/csa.shtml**.

MILK

For information about how to obtain raw milk in your state, visit the Real Milk campaign at **www.realmilk.com/where**.

California residents: You can have certified Grade A pasture-grazed raw milk delivered straight to your door from the raw dairy farm Organic Pastures, along with raw, cream, colostrum, butter, buttermilk, and more. The Frequently Asked Questions page of the farm's website is also a great source of information about raw versus pasteurized milk. For more information or to order, call **877-RawMilk (729-6455)** or visit **www.organicpastures.com**.

Flour Mills

When it comes to a home grain mill, the key is to keep the grain from heating up during the grinding, since heat accelerates oxidation of the oils in the grain. This means buying a mill with a grinding mechanism made of stone (usually the mineral corundum) as opposed to metal. You'll find more information as well as a wide selection of home grain mills to examine at **www.juicersforless.com** or **www.skippygrainmills.com.au**. In addition, we recommend the following two mills based on their superior durability and performance.

LEE HOUSEHOLD FLOUR MILLS are made by EM Lee Engineering in Milwaukee, WI, based on original designs of Dr. Royal Lee. There are four models to choose from. For more information, call **414-247-1127** or visit **www.eminstrumentswi.com/lee.html**.

GRANO 200 ELECTRIC STONE MILL BY SCHNITZER can be ordered from **www.skippygrainmills.com.au**.

About Dr. Royal Lee

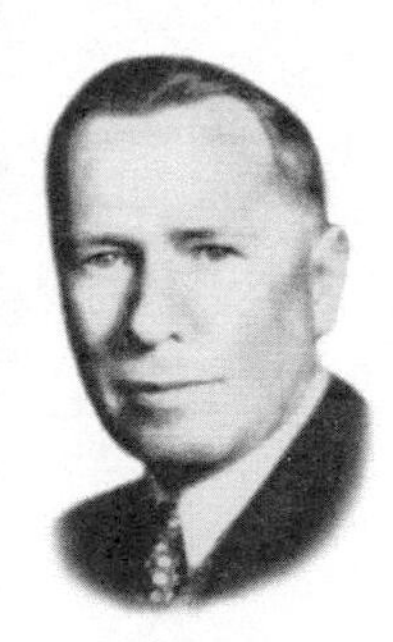
Dr. Royal Lee

In 1929, **Dr. Royal Lee** founded Vitamin Products Company, a whole-food supplement company that he eventually renamed Standard Process Laboratories.

Raised on a farm that his Norwegian grandfather settled in 1845 near Dodgeville, Wisconsin, Dr. Lee developed an interest in science and nutrition early in life, at the local elementary school. At age 12, he compiled a notebook of definitions of terms in biochemistry and nutrition, and he began collecting books on these subjects. A collection that started as a hobby continued throughout his lifetime to eventually become part of the Dr. Royal Lee Memorial Library.

After serving in the First World War, Dr. Lee graduated in 1924 from Marquette University Dental School in Wisconsin. While attending the university, his primary interest became the importance of nutrition. A paper he prepared in 1923 outlined the relationship of vitamin deficiency to tooth decay and showed the necessity of vitamins in the diet. His research led to the development of CATALYN®, a vitamin concentrate derived from whole foods. Introduced in 1929, CATALYN became the nucleus of a complete line of nutritional supplements at the Vitamin Products Company.

Dr. Lee believed the key to maintaining the quality of nutritional supplements was a unique manufacturing process. He designed high-vacuum, low-temperature drying equipment to preserve the living enzyme systems of the whole foods. These technologies continue to be used today.

From a small two-room facility, the Vitamin Products Company has evolved into the present company we call Standard Process, Inc., in Palmyra, Wisconsin. Standard Process is still family-owned and operated. Their large, certified-organic farms serve as a source for most of the whole-food supplements they manufacture, as well as a model for agricultural groups and organizations interested in learning large-scale organic farming methods. The company is continually growing, building on expert research and quality manufacturing first imposed by Dr. Lee.

In addition to working in the nutrition field, Dr. Lee was the inventor of a wide variety of dental, mechanical, automotive, and electrical equipment. He filed over 70 patents for all types of equipment, processes, internal combustion engines, and food products. For more information on Dr. Lee and Standard Process products, call **800-848-5061**, or visit **www.standardprocess.com**.

Book Series Published by Selene River Press

The Quest for Superior Nutrition Series

Put Your Money Where Your Mouth Is! A Guide to Healthy Food Shopping, by Stephanie Selene Anderson. ISBN: 978-0-9645709-4-8.

Dr. Royal Lee Library Series

Lectures of Dr. Royal Lee, Vol. I, arranged and edited by Mark R. Anderson. ISBN: 978-0-9645709-2-4.

Lectures of Dr. Royal Lee, Vol. II, compiled, edited, and audio engineered by Mark R. Anderson and Stephanie Selene Anderson. Boxed set of 32 audio CD-ROMs. ISBN: 978-0-9645709-3-1.

From Soil to Supplements: A Course in Food, Diet, and Nutrition, Taught by Dr. Royal Lee; arranged and edited by Mark R. Anderson. ISBN: 978-0-9645709-6-2.

Health Science Series

Vaccination: Examining the Record, by Judith A. DeCava, CNC, LNC. ISBN: 978-0-9645709-7-9.

Cholesterol, Facts and Fantasies, by Judith A. DeCava, CNC, LNC. ISBN: 978-0-9645709-5-5.

The Real Truth About Vitamins and Antioxidants, by Judith A. DeCava, CNC, LNC. Expanded second edition. ISBN: 978-0-9645709-8-6.

Media Titles Published by Selene River Press

Lectures of Dr. Royal Lee, Vol. II, compiled, edited, and audio engineered by Mark R. Anderson and Stephanie Selene Anderson. (From the Dr. Royal Lee Library Series above.) Boxed set of 32 audio CD-ROMs. ISBN: 978-0-964-5709-3-1.

"The Legendary Formulas of Dr. Royal Lee," presented by Dr. Michael Dobbins. Audio cassette and CD-ROM.

"The Triad: Dr. Royal Lee and the Immune System." Lecture by Mark R. Anderson. Audio CD-ROM.

"Healthy Traditional Diets." Lecture by Sally Fallon. Audio CD-ROM.

"News and Views on Nutritional Therapeutics," by Judith A. DeCava, CNC, LNC. Collection of Newsletter Articles on CD-ROM.